Bi F　　　　　n

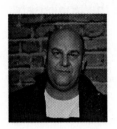

By Neil Walton

D1332418

Published by:
Chipmunka publishing
PO Box 6872
Brentwood
Essex
CM13 1ZT
United Kingdom

www.chipmunkapublishing.com

FOREWORD

WHY I WROTE THIS BOOK

After my second breakdown, Bill's wife, Seron said casually one afternoon, "Why don't you write a book about your experiences, it might help people in the same situation as yourself?" (You will get to know Bill and Seron as you read on. Bill probably saved my life, and Seron and her family were instrumental in my recovery). I dismissed the idea of writing a book as ludicrous saying, "Who would be interested in a book about me?" I didn't read books, much less write one, and besides my spelling and punctuation are crap! Three years later after my fourth nervous break-down Seron's suppressed suggestion came to the fore-front of my mind. I began jotting down notes every time the soaps were on T.V. Three months later after reading over my notes, I saw the possibilities of a short book.

I took the idea to my occupational therapist and waited for fits of raucous laughter. Hilary said simply, "Let's get you published first." I couldn't believe anybody would actually take me seriously. I joined an editorial team called *'Equilibrium,'* which produces a quarterly news letter covering mental health issues in the Haringey area. On my first day there I tentatively mentioned to the facilitator, Julia Bard that I was thinking of writing a book about being diagnosed with a bi-polar disorder. I sat back in my chair and waited for a pat on the head, followed by a bout of uncontrollable apoplexy. Julia's concise reply was, "That's a great idea, strong subject too. Bring some of your work in and I'll run it past the team. We'll edit your piece of course and use it in our next edition." Well slap me with a four pound trout! That was the first time I had heard my 'scribbling's' described as work. I didn't have a reason not to carry on writing. That was in May 1999.

In the summer of 2001 I passed my GCSE English language exam with 'C' and 'B' grades. Not bad for a forty-three year old manic depressant!

My book, Bi-Polar Expedition, turned out much bigger than I had imagined, I sincerely hope you find it useful.

Neil Walton
July 2003

THE TALE OF WOE

My childhood was a happy time in my life. My mum and dad were the best parents anyone could wish for. And a large part of my working life was spent laughing, grafting and paying the bills. In 1988 my marriage fell apart. To add to this, in 1989 I was made redundant for the first time when the printers I worked for, D.S. Colour International went into administrative receivership. Twelve years of work ended in one fell swoop one afternoon in January. Six weeks later I resumed work at another firm, only to be made redundant again four months later, a month before Christmas 1989. The icing on my cake of doom was watching my father die of lung cancer on November the 2nd 1990. It crushed my spirit to the point of attempted suicide.

Prior to this, I had been drinking heavily every night for eighteen months. I felt as if the entire structure of my life was falling apart, and so I resumed to alcohol as a way out. The worst part was not being able to control these life-altering losses. On three separate occasions I managed to find new employment, but having a mental illness meant that I was unable to sustain a working life. Eventually my flat was repossessed and I felt as if I was left with nothing. By then I had moved on from clinical depression and was diagnosed with a bi-polar disorder. I regained some, if not all of my lost marbles and today I am stabilised on Lithium and anti-depressants. Unable to return to my old trade I fell into writing by chance. I found a way of channelling my negative energy and turning it into positive thought. I simply wrote it all down onto paper... lots of it. I am a special person and I don't mind saying it out loud now. I survived everything that you are about to discover in this book...

After reading the first 70 pages I wrote my eldest son, Daniel, broke down in tears. He said, "That upset me, I didn't realise that you had been through so much." Poignantly the pages he read were about the beginning of my illness and my first hospital admission. At that stage I hadn't seen my kids for over 10 weeks. A short dad cuddled his son's six foot frame and with a lump in my throat I replied, "You were only 11 at the time mate, it all happened a long time ago." In truth, I still remember it as if it were yesterday, but at least it is in the past now.

What saddened me the most was that my disorder had raped me of my passion for music. Then it had the audacity to remove my chuckle button as well – never again! I now know that my sense of humour is one of my finest qualities.

EDUCATION IS A WONDERFUL THING

By the same token, a little knowledge can be a dangerous commodity. Please read the following quotation carefully. "I am not mad, I am not a nutter, I am not a lunatic I simply have an illness that you cannot see, and consequently you don't understand do you?"

Rest assured, if you suffer from any form of depression, sooner or later you will find that you are surrounded by people who don't understand your plight. You will get used to the blank looks when you try to explain the pain you are in. Only a sufferer or a health care specialist can sympathise with you without sounding patronising. In short, do not isolate yourself from your nearest mental health centre. Surround yourself with people who know what you are going through. If you were in traction or in a plaster cast up to your hips, things would be so much easier to explain. You would have visible evidence of your ailment. We the sufferers don't have that luxury; there is no sling for the brain. So we have to educate those around us. That was the main reason for writing this book.

You can't catch depression, it's not an airborne viral infection, but like cancer it is an invisible illness. Some people have it and die from it, but if you don't say the word, CANCER, you might not get it yourself. Both of the above illnesses still fall into the, 'don't tell the neighbours' category. This book will make you cry or at the very least put a lump in your throat. It will definitely make you laugh. But ultimately, it will help you to understand what it is like to have and survive a complete nervous break-down. Just remember, human emotions are something we all use the most in our day to day lives but we still know very little about them…

THE SLIPPING CLUTCH THEORY EXPLAINED

The car and the human being are very much alike. Both need a source of fuel to function properly. Both need regular maintenance, and from time to time they need rest and new parts. Remove the petrol from the tank and the engine won't run. Forget to put oil in, and the engine will seize up eventually. If you have a drain on your battery you will lose the positive charge. If you don't eat or sleep properly for a number of years, you're heading for trouble. Add stress to your deprivation and a copious amount of alcohol, and it is at that point that you should book an appointment with your doctor. In plain English, a nervous break-down creeps up on its victim like a slipping clutch. You use your car everyday and each time you do the clutch stretches that little bit more. Fifteen months down the line you should get it checked over, but you don't bother because it's still working. Three years later your clutch cable snaps in the middle lane of an approaching round-about!

STAMPING OUT THE STIGMA

I don't think my book will kill off the stigma attached to mental illness entirely, but I would like to think it puts a bloody great dent in it. Mention you have a flu virus at work and there will still be people in the room with you two minutes later. Openly admit you have a mental health history on your first day at a new firm and it's amazing how many people think there is a fire drill practice. Sufferers of depression don't want sympathy; we just need to be understood. Recovery from a break-down is an open ended period, and it affects different people in different ways. We don't wallow in self pity because we enjoy it. I don't sit in a confused state simply to wind my wife up, some days I just can't think straight. Depression is a fluctuating illness you see.

This book is dedicated to my mum, Jeanne and is in memory of my dad, Peter. I would also like to thank my sister, Lesley for all of the work and time that she put into this my first book.

Neil

MY MATE BILL

Bill and I go back along way, as far back as the first days of school at Chingford C of E, 1962. We did the cubs and scouts thing at different troops so our paths crossed at Gilwell Park and also at joint camping holidays. We swam and dived for the county respectively, and played in the same football team for the scout's league.

We parted company during our later years when we went to different senior schools. One morning I was standing at Chingford Station on the way to work, when I felt a tap on my shoulder, it was Bill. He had just started working for BT, and I was two years into my printing apprenticeship. We hadn't seen each other for five years; however we picked up right from where we left off. We drank together, laughed together and eventually played in the same band together. He was a talented guitarist and I was a drummer looking for a band. After the band split up we went our separate ways again. Three years had passed when quite by chance I bumped into Seron, Bill's then girlfriend. They were now married and had two sons, Ben and Sam.

At that point my marriage had dissolved, Dad was terminally ill, and I was soon too be made redundant from a long standing job. This was just the start of my turn in the barrel. I kept falling down and both Bill and Seron seemed to be there to pick me up. From the start of my clinical depression, my redundancy, and my first three nervous break-downs they were always on hand for emotional support. Over a four year period I was in their house more than I was in my own, and I never once heard them say, 'no we can't help you.'

He and Seron had their share of problems too. Bill was made redundant from BT soon after the birth of his first son. Eighteen months after their second son was born, Seron finally had to admit to herself that Sam wasn't developing as he should. It turned out that he and a group of children in the same area had been inoculated with a ineffective batch of the MMR vaccine. The years ahead were full of subdued heart ache for the pair of them. Bill's entrepreneurial skills came to the fore when he parted ways with BT to open an estate agent's. Business flourished, and this encouraged him to expand into building freelance work, which ran in parallel with his letting company. Bill's aim in life was to be a millionaire by the time he was 50. If anybody was going to achieve this, he would. However, Bill eventually sold his business interests and moved to America. Inevitably, we lost touch again. We are due to bump into each other in the near future. He joined a company that manufactured furniture for children with special needs. Bless you both and thank you for all your help in the past...

THIS YEAR'S BLACKNESS

I sit here like many condemned to this illness,
What I hadn't banked on was all the stillness.

After thirty-two years of row and noise,
I no longer felt like one of the boys.

Sitting in darkness the mind drifts away,
Suffering from years of mental decay.

Knowing tomorrow I'll feel just the same,
I'm slipping, but slowly, I'm going insane.

Neil Walton

13/9/99

CHAPTER ONE

<<<< THE LONG LIE IN >>>>

I had been on the missing list for sometime; ignoring the phone, the door and the outside world. My mind and body had taken such a battering over the past three years, (1986-89) and I just couldn't take it any more. I didn't have the energy for conversation. My brain was on overload and my body was paralysed and lethargic. I had turned into an introvert, the direct opposite of my usual character. My arms and legs were like lead and I felt bone cold, as if my core temperature was lower than any body else's. Add to that a poor diet and a feeling of utter worthlessness; I was a sorry example of a human being.

I had a loop-tape of losses and problems to come relentlessly playing in my head. The only thing that stopped this tape was sleep - the next step was obvious. I was at breaking point. If I could have laid my hands on a gun... I might not be here now. Only a fellow sufferer or a specialist would understand the mental pain I was experiencing. I found a scalpel blade in my toolbox and went into my bedroom closing the door behind me. I gazed at the sterilised *Swan & Morton* for hours on end, the loop-tape still playing. I slept most of the time. But there were those awful four to six hours spent awake, going over and over the reasons for ending my life. Why was this happening to me? What had I done to deserve this treatment from life? The answer of course was nothing.

I began nicking at the skin on my left arm just to test the pain factor. With a brand new blade it was quite painless. Then I cut deeper into my arm making seven to eight cuts between my forearm and biceps. I watched as my blood pumped from the wounds. I laid there in a cold sweat as it trickled down my arm and soaked into the duvet cover. Sometime later, I reached for my lighter and cigarettes which were on the bedside cabinet. I was momentarily prevented as the duvet cover was firmly stuck to my forearm with congealed blood. As I pulled it away from my arm, it opened four of the cuts I had inflicted on myself. I remember thinking that this wasn't going to be easy. The pain was so severe that I had to stop and think of an alternative way to end it all. The options seemed endless at the time. What about an overdose of paracetamol? How many would I have to take? If I could have been sure that I would have just gone to sleep and not woken up to being resuscitated, I might have chosen that option. As it was, I continued questioning each form of suicide but had no answers - looking back it probably saved me. My lethargy was so painfully strong that I couldn't find the energy to drag myself to the chemist, only a hundred feet from my front door. I drank a glass of water, lit another cigarette and laid there wondering what to do next.

I thought long and hard about my sons, Jack and Daniel, who I think played a key factor of my survival. How could I even think of leaving them fatherless? I felt so selfish and yet in so much pain. Suicide or death in general seems so unfair. You die and everybody who knows you suffers in one way or another. What a dilemma, what a guilt trip, as if I didn't feel bad enough already. I went back to sleep with thoughts of my parents, children and close friends on my mind.

I came to in the early hours of the morning, with tears streaming down my face I said out loud, "Oh Christ no, not another day, why can't I just die in my sleep?" You see the tape kicks in the second you're conscious. Shit, shit, shit, why was I taking this out on myself? Hours later I began to pick at the tendons on my left wrist with the blade. I wondered how long it would take to die. More importantly, how painful would it be? Would my heart simply stop? Maybe my lungs would cease functioning? How was I going to breathe? As you can see my sense of logic and reasoning was out to lunch.

My indecision was getting as bad as the loop-tape. I wanted the death part but without the pain, I should be so lucky! If I slashed my wrist I would have to cut through my tendons, something I hadn't contemplated until now. I followed a vein from my forearm to the base of my biceps with the scalpel blade. In the crease of my left arm I had a bigger target and no visible tendons. All I had to do now was push the blade in. I stabbed either side of the vein. Forty-eight hours later I was still deliberating about my attempted suicide.

I heard the third dawn chorus - you wouldn't believe the row those bloody birds made first thing in the morning. My next stop was going to be my garage, quiet and dark all the time - perfect. I guess I had it in mind to starve my self to death. If that were the case why was I contemplating taking bottles of water with me? Probably to keep my mouth and throat lubricated as I am a heavy smoker. So, with a supply of H20 and as many fags as I could carry, this being my only source of nutrition in the last seventy-two hours, the next task would have been to haul the mattress off of my bed and dump it in the garage. But I was so weak I couldn't shift it off the bed. Let alone pull it down two flights of stairs and drag it across the car park. It has been said that to take your life is the coward's way out. Yeah, bollocks it is!

What caused my suicide attempt was a catalogue of disasters one after another over a three-year period. They plunged me slowly and painfully into clinical depression. I was powerless to stop it and the last person to know I was ill.

After three days I eventually answered the door. It was Bill, a close friend and school mate of mine. "We've been concerned about you mate, so has your Mum, nobody has heard from you in a while, we just wondered if you were all right?" "Yeah, sorry mate," I replied. "I'm okay, I just feel a bit tired that's all apart from that I'm fine." I tried to make small talk to mask my real feelings but Bill saw through this like a glass book.

I couldn't keep up the pretence any longer. The smile disappeared from my face and my head fell forward into my hands. I showed him my arm. "Why am I doing this to myself Bill?" He was very calm about the situation. "You've had a lot of stress in the last three years, things that were out of your control. Basically it's affected your health."

Bill's mother-in-law had been in the nursing profession for over twenty years and saw my break-down coming. It was she who advised Bill on how to help me I later found out. The advice was simple. Without too much fuss, get Neil to his doctor, he is suffering from clinical depression. Bill's words to me were, "I think we should make a trip to the quacks, what do you reckon?" "I know I'm not a hundred percent," I said, "but is it really that serious?" He just shut his eyes and nodded a couple of times. Pre-empting my answer Bill had already phoned my GP - they were just waiting for us to arrive. "Could you take me?" I asked. "The car's outside mate," he said. "What, today? … What, now?" "When you're ready," he replied.

Bill was the sort of friend you could trust with your life. For him to be worried about me I knew I had to put my faith, what was left of it, in his judgement. I made another pot of tea, the British thing to do in a situation like this. I sat down to let the information sink in, not realising just how life-altering this visit to the doctor's was going to be.

When we arrived at the surgery the receptionist showed us straight into my doctor's room. She asked me some questions relating to diet, sleep pattern and motivation. My reply to all three was just one word, "Poor." The final question from my doctor, knowing in my heart it was rhetorical, was the hardest, shortest and the most painful I have ever had to answer. There was a terrible, sickening silence after she said the words "Have you tried to harm yourself in anyway?" "Yes," I said quietly. After that I don't remember speaking any more. I was mentally exhausted and overwhelmed with emotion. I had to let Bill take over the proceedings. He asked my GP what the next step was. Doctor Gibbon replied, "I think it would be best for Neil to see Dr. Gadhvi, the head psychiatrist at Claybury Hospital. I have made an appointment for Neil to see him this afternoon. I need a second opinion. Based on his report Neil may have to go into hospital for a short time."

Things were moving too quickly for me, with talk of head shrinks and hospitals, but I was in no fit state to argue. I was swept along with the tide after that. This was starting to feel like a sad episode of "Casualty" come to life. Karen Gibbon was a kind, caring and considerate person. She made sure I understood what was going on, without belittling me, emphasising that a stay in hospital would be probable, after my consultation with the other doctor. Family and friends had carefully planned my path towards hospital; the trip to the trick-cyclist was a mere formality.

After visiting Dr Gadhvi my fate was secured. I fell silent again. This was too much to cope with. Bill took over as my ears, eyes and brain. At the end of the consultation it was decided that I would go in hospital as a voluntary patient for a minimum of two weeks. Technically I was sectioned under the Mental Health Act, but I was informed I could leave the hospital any time I liked. Bill asked the doctor when this would happen and was told, "There will be a bed ready for him tonight. Perhaps this afternoon you could help Neil pack a bag," Bill nodded in agreement. Christ, what do I pack? I've never been in hospital before, let alone a nut house. What the fuck is it going to be like in there? Of course I had a vivid picture in my mind, who wouldn't? At this point I was petrified and powerless.

This was another situation that was totally out of my control. My life was now in other people's hands. I didn't like it one little bit. Bill was still on hand for support, and later that evening he ferried me to the hospital. It was only a short ride, but I remained quiet for hours as I remember. Communication was down to hearing and nodding only. I didn't have the strength for anything else.

As you walk through the doors of the hospital, the full magnitude of the building hits you. Streams of wide endless corridors with ceilings thirty feet high greet you. Through the interior doors I could see some of the inmates shuffling around near the entrance. There seemed to be an invisible force field keeping them inside because none of them tried to escape as you would imagine. I suddenly felt deeply embarrassed and ashamed of my predicament. In my eyes, at that point in my life, I was a total failure.

The light at the end of my tunnel had been snuffed out. Did I have to come to such a place to re-ignite it? I didn't have a choice anymore. Set in woodlands well off the beaten track, near Chigwell in Essex, the hospital had a stigma to match its size. The grade II listed building lay at the heart of an estate which covered a massive one hundred and fifty square acres of land. Built in 1893, it had been a bombproof sanctuary for the mentally ill for over ten decades. In its heyday, Claybury could care for over two thousand patients. But due to government cutbacks, this figure had been dramatically reduced to just five hundred when I was first admitted in February 1993.

The wards were marked alphabetically, A1/2 right through to Z1/2. Fifty-two wards formed a huge circle in which all the departments extended. To give a clearer idea of just how big this place was, here is a list of just some of the facilities. There was a benefits office, sub-post office, a church, laundry, path lab and a massive kitchen, a dental surgery, an E.C.T. room, a dispensary and even a hairdresser.

I followed Bill to the reception desk where he asked for directions to ward N2. As we walked down a long gloomy corridor, I felt like a condemned man going to the gallows. There was no turning back now. I was entering this place of my own accord and at some point Bill was going to walk away and leave me there. I wasn't looking forward to that all. We climbed a flight of stairs to find a large white door with a sign on it saying N2 in a bold typeface. Bill pressed the doorbell and a few moments later somebody looked through the eyepiece and then unlocked the door. This entrance led us into a large pastel blue painted hallway. There were a few seats lined up against the wall, with a battered looking phone on it. When some of the inmates spied two bits of fresh meat walking in, we became an immediate target for requests for cigarettes. A small group of patients were talking at the tops of their voices about things that made no sense at all. The nurse didn't bat an eyelid. Obviously this was the ward norm, or abnormality as the case may be. Was this the real twilight zone?

Bill told the nurse my name and he showed us to a table next to the ward office. "Right," he said. "Your name is Neil Walton." "Yes," I replied. He asked for my home address then proceeded to ask me a number of questions relating to how I was feeling at that particular moment in time. I told him, "I felt tired, freezing cold and just a little scared to death." He asked me if I knew where I was. "Yes," I replied with a lump in my throat. "I'm in Claybury Hospital." "Do you know why you are here Neil?" "I'm here to get better." I answered pathetically. He went on, "Some of these questions may seem a little strange but they will help us to determine your mental state at the present time." "Do you feel like harming yourself or anybody else?" "No," I replied. "Have you tried to harm yourself in the past?" "Yes."

The next question took me by surprise. The nurse asked me if I had heard voices in my head. I thought about it momentarily, not wishing to give him the impression I had. I then replied as nonchalantly as I could saying, "No." I had of course listened to my Dad's voice, which to me was quite normal, as he had not long passed over. I have had a lot of psychic occurrences in my life that I would still like explained to me. However, this all happened when I was mentally healthy, so I was buggered if I was going tell a complete stranger working in a psychiatric hospital that I had heard voices. I would have never been discharged. I felt as though I had used my last remaining marbles wisely.

I felt my Dad's presence when I wrote the first draft of these pages. It was 4.00 a.m. and the rain was pouring down the windows. It was still dark, and the ticking clock in my room was the only thing that broke the silence. Sometimes I can feel him with me, which gives me a great sense of well-being and strength. I thought the signing-in procedure was nearly over and Bill must have had enough of hanging around. We had been in the hospital well over an hour by now. Once the paperwork had been dealt with I was shown to my sleeping quarters. I wasn't impressed with the thought of sharing my bed space in a dormitory with 26 inmates. There were clothes strewn over a big radiator and two patients were already asleep. One of them was snoring like a bull elephant. The only privacy you had was a thin cotton curtain that hung between each bed from a rail.

We were shown into the day room. At one end, near a huge bay window, was a table tennis table. In the centre of the room there were thirty armchairs, with some small tables scattered around. Most of them had dirty tin foil ashtrays on them, half of which were filled with hand rolled cigarette butts. We sat down again and I now had to give the nurse a list of my clothing in case anything was stolen during my stay. Bill was ever so patient while this was going on, I was so glad he was with me.

It was a terrible day for me; I couldn't have coped without him. Once my clothes had been accounted for the nurse said, "That's almost it, you just have to be checked over by a duty doctor." Bill was about to leave. He gave me a long hug and said, "Don't forget, Seron and I will be thinking of you and we will come and visit you as soon as we are allowed to." His final comment was, "Take good care of yourself, love ya," and with that he left. I fought hard to stop myself from crying. I heard the heavy door shut behind him, and a few seconds after that the door was locked. I was now friendless and terrified of my first night in a psychiatric hospital and dreading the next full day.

The last hurdle I had to face was the visit from the duty doctor. I sat down smoking cigarette after cigarette. Half an hour must have past by when I saw a youngish man walk into the ward office. I presumed he was the duty doctor. A few minutes later the nurse introduced him to me and he asked me to follow him into a small side room. He took my blood pressure and then checked my breathing. Then he started to prod my liver about, asking me questions as he went about his examination.

"Do you smoke?" "Yes," I said. "Drink?" He asked coldly. "Yes," I replied. "Taken drugs?" He inquired harshly. "I smoked cannabis about fifteen years ago if that counts." "Okay, that's it," he said. It was all over in five minutes. I didn't much care for his bedside manner. I was glad when it was all over. I felt as though I had ruined his evening. By the way he was dressed it looked as if he had to break off a dinner date or a night at the opera.

At 7.30 p.m. I was introduced to an agency nurse called Lenny. He took me down to the tearoom and gave me a run down of the daily routine in the hospital. It was difficult to make conversation with him, mainly because of the bloody row coming from some of the other patients. Most of the guys involved looked like extras that had been rejected from the Michael Jackson video, Thriller. It was a woeful sight this place, it really was, and a huge culture shock to me. Unless you have ever visited a mental hospital you can't fully appreciate just how terribly sad places like these are. I had been plucked out of public life for my own health and safety, and voluntarily signed myself into this hellhole.

At eight o'clock Lenny took me back to the ward. The door was locked behind us. I asked him why it was locked. He said, "It was a standard security procedure." I remember thinking at the time, whose security? Who in their right mind would try breaking into this place? I went back into the day room and sat down to survey my new surroundings. I didn't like what I saw. There was a bunch of what looked like child molester's playing cards at one of the tables. A nurse and a patient playing table tennis, and at the other end of this huge room, were a group of Charles Manson look-a-likes playing darts. What prat gave them a set of pointy sharp things!?! One of them piped up, "I've got implants in my head you know. The Russians put them in there!" Oh fuck, I could see it was going to be one of 'those' nights. None of the people on the ward looked capable of offering up much in the way of stimulating conversation, except for the staff of course.

The toilets reeked of cheap pungent cleaning fluid, the bathroom was cold and uninviting, and my bedroom had no privacy whatsoever. My bed was hard and the mattress was covered in plastic, in case of an incontinent patient. The sheets were thick, starched and cold and the pillows were uncomfortably big. To round off this five star accommodation for the mentally challenged; my bed had a blanket on it that wouldn't have kept a baby warm, let alone an adult. I could see I wasn't going to get much sleep on my first night in the slammer.

The staff on my ward did their best to help me settle into the daily routine of hospital life. I had already been put on anti-depressants, but after four days I wanted to know why I didn't feel any better? I asked the nurse in charge of the medication why the tablets were not working. He answered with a smile, "Don't worry, they take two to four weeks to get in your system." They've got me now, I thought, my fourteen-day sentence had just doubled in the time it took to swallow a tablet. I've seen this scenario before somewhere; the only things missing were the men in white coats. I wished I'd never asked the bloody question in the first place. I couldn't help feeling as though I had been ganged up on. Now I was scared to ask any more questions in case my stay in the funny farm was extended any further. I was thirty-three years of age but I felt like a frightened child who had just lost his mum in the high street.

On day five I was informed I would soon begin a course of E.C.T. "Oh great!" I exclaimed, "I can hardly wait." Gingerly I asked what E.C.T. stood for. I just knew it was going to be something I didn't like the sound of. "Electro-convulsive therapy," the nurse replied. See what I mean! "Well, I'm okay with the therapy part," I said, "but I'm not to chuffed with the words 'convulsive' or 'electro.'" It sounded too much like a Hammer House of Horror film. Trisha, the head nurse on the day shift, did her best to reduce my doubts about this form of treatment. She then proceeded to tell me one step at a time, how E.C.T. is administered to patients. Trish took her time explaining the process, and answered all of my questions to settle my nerves. Even so I still went away with a nagging fear in the back of my mind. (Why do we say that? Is the cerebellum where all of my worrying starts?).

The fateful day arrived. A group of us assembled outside the ward office. We were led down a maze of poorly lit corridors towards the E.C.T. room. We looked like a bunch of P.O.W's being taken down to the cells to be experimented on by the SS. We were shown into a small blue painted waiting room, just big enough to seat all twelve of us. A few silent moments had passed by, when a nurse came in with a small hot water bottle for each of us. "That's very nice of you," I said "but I couldn't eat another thing thanks!" She smiled and explained that they were for us to keep our hands warm. The heat makes your veins stand up which gives the anaesthetist something to aim at, before she puts you under. Still smiling, she disappeared back into the E.C.T. room. So there we sat, the lucky dozen crammed into a room the size of a rabbit hutch, all waiting with bated breath for a swift surge of the National Grid!

One member of the group piped up, "I wonder if we'll get charged for this on our next electricity bill?" Needless to say, we all had a bloody good laugh at this bloke's sharp wit. That was the first time I had cracked a smile in ten months. To have lost my sense of humour was heartbreaking for me; I now know it's one of my finest qualities. Most of us in that room couldn't boil an egg, let alone crack a joke (pun unintended.) Yet faced with a largely unknown situation, we all did our best to make humorous small talk to pass the time. I now know it's the brain's natural defence mechanism against blind fear.

Our names were being called out every ten minutes. Now there were just five of us left, and the small-talk had all but diminished. We all sat there starring vaguely into space waiting for our turn. Then I heard my name called. "Oh shit," I thought, "here we go," and a nurse led me into the E.C.T. room. It was large and brightly lit. Inside five other nurses were laughing and talking to each other. It wasn't quite the Nazi torture chamber that I had envisaged.

In fact it had a nice calming effect on me. For the first time that day, I slowly began to relax. The nurse that brought me in asked if I would like another run through of the treatment. I said, "Yes please." She was so understanding and kind, and could see that I was scared stiff. The explanation of the treatment is a lot easier to take in with all of the equipment in front you. "Are you ready?" She asked. "Not really," I replied nervously. "It will be fine, honestly," still trying to reassure me. "Come on then," I said, "let's get it over with." "Okay, first take off your shoes and socks and then lay on the bed Neil. I will take you through it one step at a time." At this point the other nurses gathered around the four corners of my bed. They carried on talking away as if they were down the supermarket. On reflection, it was this bedside manner that put me at ease with the situation I now found myself in. There wasn't a dull face in the room, except mine of course.

"You will feel a slight jab in your hand," the nurse said, "that's the needle going in for the anaesthetic. You will be asleep for about ten minutes. While you're under, I will place some electrodes on each temple and give you a measured shock of electricity. This throws your brain into an epileptic fit." Oh, I could hardly contain myself. "The nurses around you will prevent you from putting any joints out of place by holding down your limbs as your body convulses." Sounds like a wonderful experience doesn't it! "Here we go - ready?" I winked at her and took a sharp intake of breath as the needle punctured the skin and vein on the back of my left hand.

"You will feel a cold sensation creeping up your arm. That's the anaesthetic going in. In about ten seconds you will be under." Within two seconds the anaesthetic had already reached my elbow and had started to affect my vision. It was a pleasant feeling I have to say. I tried desperately to keep my eyes open, saying to the nurse, "I'm going to try and stay awa…" I never finished the sentence - it was lights out.

When you come to your senses, you are in the recovery room wondering how the hell you got there. Come to think of it, I couldn't remember where I was before either. And why did I take my shoes and socks off? In the distance I could hear people talking and the chink of cups on saucers. A nurse came to check on me. I was still a bit woozy after the anaesthetic. As I came round she warned me not to stand up to quickly, in case I fell over. "When you come round a bit more you can join the others for a drink."

My throat was as dry as a yak's armpit. All I wanted now was a gallon of tea and twenty cigarettes. I sat up, looked around, found my trainers and socks and put them on as quickly as I could. I was gagging for something to drink. In my haste I had forgotten what the nurse had said. I stood up and promptly fell back towards the bed. I panicked. I couldn't work out why my arms and legs wouldn't function properly. I sat back for a few minutes and tried hard to retrace my steps, but all I could remember was being knocked out - the rest was a total blank.

I got up, slower this time, and walked into the tea-room like an OAP who had just taken six Valium. I was beaming from ear to ear. The only drawback, it seemed was a skull-splitting headache. Everybody was in the same state. I saw faces I knew but couldn't recall their names and like me, none of them could remember what had just happened. Yet we all sat there grinning at each other like Cheshire cats. My bloody cheeks were killing me afterwards. The jolt of electricity had jump-started my brain into happy mode. I couldn't believe the change in myself.

We went back to the ward and started queuing for painkillers. As the day wore on the headaches subsided and the enforced smiling stopped. A few of us sat down and talked about what we had just been through. We had all experienced some form of memory loss. I couldn't remember my date of birth for example. It was frightening to think that something like that could be erased from my memory. I was glad I wasn't the only one feeling like it, something to do with safety in numbers I suppose. Days after the treatment, I was still having trouble remembering things, but E.C.T. had definitely shifted my morose mood to a euphoric state at the flick of a switch. I had six sessions of E.C.T. followed by what can only be described as intermittent amnesia. I was discharged from Claybury Hospital after one month and was in a better frame of mind, though I was still suffering the side-effects of my medication and the E.C.T. memory block. I will cover the side effects of medication in another chapter.

The side-effects of electro-convulsive therapy are headaches, initially followed by short-term memory loss. In my case, this lasted three months. On the positive side, it shifted my mood in conjunction with anti-depressants. My only concern was that the doctors were unsure of its success in lifting depression. Another possible draw back was that a maximum of sixteen sessions were allowed. If it failed to work after sixteen times then another solution would have to be found. Nobody has told me why or what happens if you have more? Interestingly enough when E.C.T. was first used fifty years ago, no anaesthetic was used. This makes me wonder, if it were to be invented today, would the British Medical Counsel allow its use in treating people suffering from clinical depression? There is no evidence of any permanent side effects caused from E.C.T.

CHAPTER TWO

<<<< HEADING FOR BREAK-DOWN No.2 >>>>

I don't remember too much of what happened after I left Claybury to be honest with you. I think Mum was in the process of selling the family home and moving to Berkhamsted. I didn't want her to move, but I didn't want to stand in her way either. This was Mum and Dad's retirement plan, had he lived. Mum had always lived a long way from her sister, Rene, since they both married. After a lifetime of parenting and work she deserved to do what she wanted for a change. When she went it was awful. Mum, Dad and the family home had been in the same place for twenty-eight years. I lived in that house from the age of four. I had moved out a few times, as did my sister, but I always had a secure base if anything went wrong. I know Mum was racked with guilt for months after moving, and I did try to alleviate some of her worry, but all the same I felt as though I had lost an arm and a leg in the same day.

I carried on taking my medication, but after a while it didn't seemed to be doing much good. A new drug had just hit the market and my GP thought it might help my mood - *it was called Prozac*. I can see now why it was called 'the sunshine drug.' I took one capsule and by the next morning I couldn't stop smiling. It worked as quickly as E.C.T., only without the storming headache that followed each session. I felt so good I began drinking again, every night for six months. By that time I thought I had escaped the clutches of my depression. I was firing on all cylinders, with both oars in the water, head facing forwards at last, and it was legal! However, this falsehood was to cause major problems in the coming months. I was heading for a bout of powerful psychotic highs. I wasn't overly confident to begin with, but as the weeks passed I remember feeling pumped all of the time, and up for anything. My razor sharp wit had returned and I was making people laugh. Everybody around me thought I was back to my old self.

Prior to my redundancies, and on Bill's advice, I had taken out an insurance policy that protected my mortgage against unemployment and illness. More importantly it covered mental illness. Bill acted on my behalf when the time came. I didn't think that the company would pay out such a vast sum of money per month without a fight, even though I fitted the policy's requirement to the letter. Bill made the call and I sat with bated breath waiting to hear their technical cop-out clause. Call me pessimistic but I was right. I checked the small print in the pamphlet and couldn't spot it, neither could Bill. He looked through the policy under a microscope and found the problem in the fine print, where else. The clause stated that I had to have paid a minimum of six months' subscriptions from a source in my profession before my claim could be validated. This excluded benefit payments. I had made four monthly payments when I was working and two payments from my benefits.

Seron said, "Don't worry, he'll think of something." Bill went quiet for a good ten minutes; lifting up his head he said with a smile, "Got it!" It was true to say that I had only made four of the six payments. All that was checkable from the date on my benefit claim form. But not only was I receiving state benefits, I was also entitled to gratuity from my union's unemployment fund. Therefore I had been paid a sum of money from my trade of work six months in a row. The policy didn't state a specific amount, but I can bet it does now. Bill got on the phone and relayed his findings. After a while the guy on the other end realised that he had been painted into a corner by the better man. "You can relax now," Bill said putting down the receiver "You're covered for 12 months; the beers are on you I think." I planted a kiss on his forehead and told him what a star he was, mentioning that if he and Seron wanted another child, I would have it for them minus the conception part!

I went for a few interviews prior to the usual fight for my benefits and eventually I took a job in a family-run print firm near the Barbican. After the spaciousness of D. S. Colour I was about to find out that size really does matter. My new department was situated below ground level and right next door to the machine room. I have never worked in a room that had it own weather system before! It was hot, dusty and noisy in the summer and damp, dusty and noisy during the winter months. More importantly there was no access for natural daylight, all of which didn't affect me to begin with.

The room itself measured approximately 18' x 12' x 10', which sounds a fair size until you put two people in it and all of the printing equipment. We had a large camera that we used to copy base artworks from. This had two powerful lamps on it and was situated in a 6 x 4 darkroom. Just outside of the sweat box was a printing down frame. This consisted of a 3 x 4 rubber backed base with a glass top. Underneath was a vacuum; this held the films and plates in a fixed position. Over head was an artificial ark lamp; this exposed our film images to the printing plates. Just to add a little extra warmth to the hamsters' maze we had the bonus of the firms' boiler pipes just above our heads. On a good month we could grow cucumbers! I had been used to working in a large open-plan room with at least eight people. Here, if you didn't get on with the person you were working with you were stuffed; there was nowhere else to go. After ten months of working in the rat run, the non-conducive atmosphere was beginning to take its toll on my health.

My new work chum didn't have the same sense of humour as I did, which was a problem for me. Soon after I started my new job he told me he was the boss's son. This news unfortunately reached me three days too late. In the pub after my first day, a member of the office staff asked me what I thought of the place. Having said what I had said I don't think I had told them anything they didn't already know. I replied, "It's dingy, cramped and to fucking hot, and the wages are crap as well, but it beats signing on." Up the workers! You can't blame a bloke for telling it like it is! Dad would have been proud of me.

I returned to my doctors and asked for my medication to be changed, as I felt too high most of the time. But I think it was too late by then, the Prozac and drink had done its damage. So it was back to a standard anti-depressant and its side-effects. This was fine for a while, until I woke up one morning with the old familiar black cloud hanging over me again. As you're probably aware there seems to be a vast difference in side-effects depending on which drugs you are prescribed. If you are not happy with the drugs you are taking, go back to your doctor and ask for them to be changed. Don't stay on something if it's making you feel odd. (This is the only way I can describe the 'vague feeling of being unwell,' printed on the paperwork in most anti-depressant packets.) This can just as easily fuck up your life in the same way that a nervous breakdown does.

I was showing signs of cracking under pressure at work. I was losing the ability to concentrate and I felt tired all of the time. My confidence was fast diminishing also. The timing couldn't have been worse for me. Five months into the job I was asked if I would go on a shift rota. I was in a tenuous position financially and felt obliged to agree to my line manager's demands. I was still biting the bullet regarding spilling the beans about my first nervous break-down. The shift required was a week of lates and a week of early's. Things were okay to begin with, but after a few months I found it harder and harder to cope. Until one night I sat in front of a job, when everybody had gone home, for three hours not knowing where to start. My work chum wasn't best pleased the next day.

He wasn't just angry, he was seething. I tried frantically to explain, but he had an answer for everything and I didn't. I'm sure you can imagine the atmosphere in the minuscule room. I could feel waves of hate washing over me for most of the morning. After that one incident I was scared stiff of making any other mistakes. My work partner seemed fine as long as everything went his way. I suppose there is something to be said for nepotism. All the same I had never encountered such hostility over a poxy four colour job before.

It hadn't occurred to me that a different shift would affect my mental state. I had worked on day shifts for over seventeen years up until that point. But the change in working nights affected my sleep pattern from week to week, which in turn affected my eating cycle. Consequently I drifted into a series of high and low episodes. Eventually after being a pain in the arse for months, I came down to earth with an almighty bang.

My boss gave me a month off to sort myself out, but I was too far gone by then. In the end I asked to be made redundant. The highs only got higher after that; I called this period, the 'walking on water' stage. At some point during my well months, I stupidly reduced my medication, over a three-month period, without my doctors' knowledge. Don't even contemplate trying this.

Prior to all of my stays in hospital there was always an abundance of incidences leading up to admission. This was largely due to the Mental Health Act of 1983, which roughly states, that unless a person is a danger to themselves or others, they can't be picked up by the old bill and carted off to the nearest fun factory. On this spree of events Mum, Bill and Seron helped to fill in the blank spaces of my second admission into Claybury Hospital.

Mum was coming over to see me knowing I wasn't quite the whole nine yards again. My sleep pattern was all over the shop, and I had stopped eating. On this particular Saturday morning, I had phoned Bill begging him and his wife, Seron to come down to my flat. The night before, I had painstakingly re-assembled my drum kit in my front room. For some reason I had decided to do this in the pitch dark at about 3.00 a.m., don't ask why, I haven't a clue. I was doing everything in slow motion at that point; I believed my patience was being tested in some way.

Normally it would take me forty minutes or so to put my kit together, but on this occasion the conditions were far from normal. I had it in my head that my flat was bugged. To add to my dilemma, I had to take each piece of equipment from a back bedroom, up the creaking hallway and into the front-room. Rhyme, reason and time-scale had abandoned me yet again, save the odd glance at the clock. It took me over two and a half hours to put up my drum kit, which I managed to do in near silence. Bill and Seron arrived about mid-day. They were visibly taken aback by the sight that had met their eyes. They were equally surprised to see that I had taken the mattresses off the bunk beds and was now using them as sound-proofing.

Bill and I had played together in a band for a number of years. He was the guitarist. One of our high-points was a Radio 1 session on the Janice Long show. The creative buzz that I had all those years ago had returned and, three months prior to this, I had blown the dust off my sticks and begun to practise again. Of all the music I listened to, one song held my attention, 'Seven Days', by Sting. It's a peach of a track in 7/8 time, and after weeks of warming up to 4/4 music it became the only song I would play.

Initially I sat for hours listening to the track as a whole, and then gradually broke the drum-patterns down into sections. Once I had the bass and snare firmly fixed in my mind, I concentrated on the cymbal pushes and finally I worked on all of the drum-fills. The only part I couldn't perfect was a short section just before the song fades out; the drummer does too many fills for my little head to remember. Now all I wanted to do was play it at the proper volume and see if I could still hack it as a drummer.

Bill and Seron sat and listened dutifully as I cranked up the stereo and put the tape on. I played the song once, and once only, using my speakers as a make-shift fold back system. One to the left of me standing on a stool and the other, to my right, angled up at forty-five degrees at the base of my Hi- hat stand. When the track finished I said out loud, "Still got it." That single performance was all the gratification I needed or expected. The next couple of hours were spent rifling through my record and tape collection reminiscing.

At 2.00 p.m. Mum arrived to find Bill, Seron and myself knee-deep in vinyl, cassettes and album covers. "What's all this then?" She asked. Seron assured her that there had only been one floor-show that afternoon. "Just as well really," she replied starring at me in disbelief. "What must have the neighbours thought?" "Sod the neighbours," I said. Unfortunately my words opened up Mum's entire book of stock phrases, volume one. Starting with, "Well that's all right for you to say," and ending with, "And another thing, did you think about that?" By the time she had gone through her entire repertoire, I had made a sandwich, eaten it and poured her out a cup of coffee. This was the only way to stop her drifting into her second volume of nagging for the Home Counties North, advanced level.

After Bill and Seron left my buzzed up mood took a dive. Poor Mum, she had only been there five minutes and already I was asking her to give me some space. Having the patience of a saint she went to visit and old friend of hers, knowing full well it would give her the opportunity to speak to my GP. Doctor Gibbon's advice to my mother was, "Go home Jeanne and give Neil the space he has asked for." I did feel embarrassed when Mum told me later what she had said. That after-noon Mum travelled back to Berkhamsted, saying she would be in touch. My guardian angel, Bill, had said to Mum he would keep an eye on me, which put her mind at rest.

Later that day Bill popped into see how I was. It's just as well he did. I was on a downer and very confused. "Why don't we go and see your doctor," he asked. "Would you come with me?" "Yeah, no problem." He replied. I think because I heard the word doctor, I recall asking him if he could drive as slowly as he could. I think it was because I was in no rush to go back in the 'fun palace.' Doctor Gibbon had opened the surgery on this Saturday afternoon to see me personally. Now that's what I call a National Heath Service. I was in such a state of confusion, apparently, that when she asked a question I drifted off mentally. I can vaguely remember mumbling away to myself as I sat cross-legged on the doctor's couch.

She gave me a large red tablet to take. This was to stop me getting any higher throughout the rest of the day. She also gave Bill a second tablet in a brown envelope for me to take at 9.00 p.m. that evening. Bill said he would make sure I took it. The whole week-end felt surreal, even more so after taking the medication. What a result, my doctor's being open on a Saturday! I really was a punnet short of a strawberry that day. Doctor Gibbon asked me if there was anything else I needed or wanted.

I thought for a moment, this being the only question I actually understood, and said, "Well, I could do with, a good, hard, shag." In complete control and with only a hint of a smile she replied, "I'm afraid we don't that on the N.H.S." At the time I was totally oblivious as to just how funny that must have sounded. Months later Bill reminded me of what I had said and we fell about laughing. It was nice to know that I still had the ability to make people laugh.

I lost the rest of Saturday and the majority of Sunday to the powerful medication I was given. Bill contacted my Mum to explain what had happened at the surgery. She was back on my door-step the very next day. I had completely lost the plot this time. For reasons best known to me I decided to put some of my tools in the washing machine and turn it on. Can you imagine the noise! God knows how long they were in there clanking around before Mum switched it off. I, of course, was totally oblivious to the row, thanks to the high I was on. From what I can gather, the best way to describe how I acting was to watch a four year old child at play.

As usual I had lost all concept of time, and was totally reliant on other people. It's a wonder I didn't start a fire, as I smoke. I guess I had a taste of what some people would like to experience again, a second child-hood. It's a shame I can't remember more of those seventy-two hours, perhaps its better I can't. I sometimes wish, when I hit a low spot, the whole twelve years of my illness had been like that lost weekend. As it is, I will remain mentally scared for the rest of my life.

I awoke with a start early on Monday morning after having a nightmare. I had dreamt that I saw my Mum was dying. She looked surprised to see me presenting her with a cup of tea but I wasn't to know it was half-past-five in the morning. I gave a sigh of relief to see my little Mum was still breathing. The next twelve hours were hectic to say the least.

Prior to Mums' arrival I had become obsessed with colour co-ordinating my clothes, all of which I separated to those of the armed forces, from khaki through to navy blue. I put the trousers on hangers followed by the shirts and then their jackets. Any other tops or T-shirts that were left over I rolled up as you would a flag and placed them on a work-top next to the kitchen sink. At this point everything had to be spotlessly clean and tidy; I also polished all of my shoes and boots, putting clean socks in each pair. I had stumbled into another fantasy, now believing that whatever colour top I had on in the morning was the service I had secretly been drafted into. If I saw someone in the street with a similar colour scheme as mine they were also in the same force. Because this would have been a hush-hush operation, I was left to guess as to what rank the other people held. On this one particular day I had put on a white T- shirt and a pair of navy blue jogging bottoms. I was convinced I was a Naval rating who had been granted shore leave. So where would I go with my imaginary forty-eight hour pass? That's right, the nearest grog shop.

Days earlier I had finger-knitted a wrist-band made from white string. This was something my dad had taught me to do as a boy. Basically, it was a means of shortening a length of rope. I just adapted it for my own purposes. I tore off a segment from a matchbox and wrapped it around a solitary match. Then I poked it through the plaited twine. As I pulled the wrist-band back into shape the string gripped my make-shift source of ignition. With this in place I turned the band around so the match and its wrapping faced my wrist and just touched the palm of my hand.

My reason for this elaborate process was obvious, but of course only to me. Although I was on shore-leave it occurred to me that I may be called upon to do a four-hour watch, well you would wouldn't you? Christ knows where of course, the nearest ship was bloody miles away. Still you never know somebody might have gone down with scurvy on HMS Belfast! Anyway I wasn't going out without a fag on me, so I tucked one behind my ear. I was in a world of my own, where it seemed my subconscious had overridden my conscious mind. I can't even remember where my Mum was before I went walk-about. I do however recall my personality changing from a serious mood to a jovial one and back again, as if someone had flicked a light-switch on.

At this juncture my imaginary furlough began to merge with a new fantasy. In my head, clear as a bell, I heard the voice of Paul McKenna the hypnotist. I was now under his control, something that was to occur again. Not only could I hear him, I could even feel the weight of his arm through mine as he led me into the car park of the flats where I lived. "Hold up," I said, "where are we going?" "Oh, just a little stroll," he replied smugly. "But I don't want to go for a walk thanks." I said in disbelief. "Well just try and stop yourself then," he answered with a chortle. So I tried to turn round, my upper body moved but my feet were firmly stuck to the pavement. The fantasy hypnosis was incredibly powerful. Try as I might I couldn't break free from its grip. I heard Paul say, "Okay, okay, I'll give you a sporting chance. After the count of three I'll release your feet, ready, one... two... three..."

My calf muscles felt as though I had just got over a bad attack of pins and needles and were slow in response to my brain's signal to move. I took a second glance at my feet and noticed I was wearing my moccasin slippers instead of my usual trainers. "Why did I put these on?" I exclaimed to an invisible Mr McKenna. "I told you to put them on," he gleefully explained. "Oh smart move," I replied sarcastically. "My feet are going to get soaked, it's started raining. What the hell is going on and why are you here? Is this some sort of a test?"

"You could call it that," he replied calmly, "and you know you're up against the best don't you." "So this is really happening is it?" I asked indignantly. "Very much so," came the reply. "Oh, and I forgot to mention, we're being filmed by Channel 4." "So where's the film crew then?" I asked. "Invisible, but only to you," came the retort.

By now I was well past the pissed off stage. I said to Paul, "I think we had better call a halt to this right now. I'm not doing anything or going anywhere I don't want to. This stops right now. I feel bad enough about myself on a good day. I don't need to be made a fool of in public like this."

After my speech of disapproval, the now not so smug, Mr McKenna could tell I wasn't a happy bunny. I had a double dose of nicotine while I listened to Paul apologise profusely. Reluctantly, I agreed to carry on with the charade. "Three…two…one… you're under," he said. "What now," I asked. "All you have to do is stop yourself from walking where I take you." I felt the weight of his hand on my shoulder and with that, both my legs from the knees downwards turned to lead. "Still want to go and get your trainers?" Paul inquired. "Yeah why not."

It was as if he was turning up the intensity of the hypnosis. I hated to admit it but I couldn't move. The leaden feeling crept up to my waist and was making a B-line for my chest. "It's a lot easier if you go with it," Paul said. We walked towards the main road and turned left at the traffic lights. The hill we were about to ascend towards was just under a mile in length, with a gradient of 1 in 3. The climb was always worth it though. At the top, stood a sight for sore eyes and a parched throat, the King's Head. With the rain still falling from the grey clouds, we began our ascent. I can vividly recall talking, giggling and swapping jokes with Paul. By the time we reached the pub, my clothes and footwear were sopping wet.

Once inside the lounge bar, I made myself at home placing my drenched moccasins in front of the open coal fire. I sunk my left hand deep into my damp pocket, only to find a small amount of fluff and a solitary penny. "Oh fine." I muttered under my breath. Not only was I minus my packet of cigarettes, I didn't have any beer vouchers either. I then remembered the snout I had placed behind my ear. I reached up to get it. All that remained of my soggy cigarette was the filter, and a few strands of wet tobacco. I felt the side of my neck, only to find the rest of my nicotine parcel had left a trail down to the neck of my T-shirt and beyond. "Oh bollocks," I mumbled to myself through gritted teeth.

As I sat down at a table near the fire I noticed a young bloke wearing a sharp, dark blue suit. He was opening a packet of Benson and hedges, "Excuse me," I said hopefully, "you couldn't spare one of those could you?" The Thatchers' grandchild looked me up and down and said, "No I can't." Jumped up little shit. I could have slapped him. I wouldn't have asked if I wasn't desperate. Perhaps I didn't look desperate enough.

My eternal pub triangle or the reason for being there, what ever that was, now had no sides to it. No cigarettes and no money equalled no beer. This stage of the afternoon had just hit the boring zone. There was no doubt in my mind that I had to re-evaluate my position. For a start, the wonderful Mr McKenna had buggered off without a trace. No hint of a kiss my arse, goodbye, nothing.

I couldn't ask the barman if he could see an invisible film crew, he was giving me funny looks as it was. Why was I here anyway? This was beginning to feel like a bad joke at my expense. I felt a floating sensation wash over me and things didn't seem so bad. I walk over to the fruit machine and put my penny in the slot. Through my eyes at least it looked as though I had won the £20 jackpot. Beer and cigarettes flashed from my brain's memory department like a May Day call. I pushed the collect button but something was missing. It was the old familiar sound of clanky bits of loose change hitting the pay out tray. I looked back up at the screen to see my winnings had vanished. This was turning out to be, 'one of those days.' This is something that still happens to me today but thankfully not so frequently. I have learnt to cope with the start of feeling high.

I run through a mental checklist: Have I missed my medication? Have I eaten? When did I last have a beer? When my mouth is working thirty six times faster than my brain, it's time to sit down and eat something. Half an hour later my blood's sugar level has balanced out. My smoking pattern slows down and my caffeine consumption is drastically reduced. Then instead of doing seven things at once, I return to the tried and tested method of, one thing at a time.

I retrieved my coin from the reject slot and took a seat next to a bearded man who was parked on a bench seat near the fire. I asked him if he could spare me some wedge for half a Guinness. "I can't do the drink," he answered, "but your more than welcome to a roll-up." "Oh cheers mate; you're a life-saver." By now I was getting that uneasy feeling you get when you know people are starring at you. So I walked to the end of the bar where there were no customers. I sat on a bar stool wondering what to do next. Oddly enough, the thought of going home didn't enter my head.

As I looked behind the bar I noticed some long stemmed champagne glasses above the optics. They had been arranged like a coconut shy but I didn't have a ball, well not as such. Although I was on an abnormal high I was still able to judge distance and height. My grey matter was sifting information, albeit over a trivial task. I was too close to the glass target area to throw my intended missile. Somehow for, reasons best known to myself, I was intent on making up a challenge. My prize, a single shot at the glass coconut shy.

I placed my penny on the floor just behind the bar stool. Then I hooked both of my feet under the foot rail that circled the bar. Sitting in an upright position, I leant over backwards to see if I could pick up the coin. It was surprisingly easy, now for the real test of strength; could I pull myself back up? I felt every muscle in my torso tense up and the blood was pounding around my head. With my feet still anchored, I raised my body back up to the bar in one slow, meticulous movement. I have to say I had impressed myself with my abdominal power. Now it was time to pick up my prize.

My problem was how to launch my projectile without throwing it, because I felt that would have been far too easy. I went through various combinations, finalising them down to three choices. I could have tried to spit the coin from where I sat. Then I thought how messy and inaccurate this might be. My second plan was to flick the penny off the back of my hand. After some careful deliberation I realised that this idea would be less accurate than my first ploy. The third option to my mind had the best chance of a successful strike rate. In front of me at the bar was a large ashtray with a hollow interior. I placed the copper coin into it and pushed it around with my forefinger and thumb. It glided from side to side quite freely, offering little resistance against the enamel surface. The angle of the hollow was roughly 35 degrees from the centre of the ashtray up to the outer rim. I had a missile, a launch pad and now the use of elevation. What I was still searching for was a means of propulsion. This whim of probability was turning into a full-scale experiment. I wrestled with the physics of what would seem too trivial for anybody else to be bothered with.

I over-lapped my forearms and placed them on the bar. Resting my chin on the back of my left hand, I pondered on how I would complete this, to me at least, important test. At this point the ashtray was right under my nose. As I exhaled I heard the coin wobble against the shiny surface. I blew out of my mouth; to my surprise I made the penny rattle from one side of the launch pad to the other. The problem now was with the coin laying flat I didn't have much of a surface area to blow against. I seemed to solve one problem, only to be faced with another.

As a true Gemini I get bored easily. I was beginning to wonder whether using all of this brain power was worth the effort. For something that was so futile, I had become totally obsessed with finding a solution. I took a breather from my experiment and wished I hadn't. While I was occupied the craving for a cigarette had subsided. All I could concentrate on now was getting hold of some nicotine. I scanned the bar like a laser, looking for new, unsuspecting customers. No such luck, it was just me, the barman, two blokes leaning on the bar and the old man who gave me the roll-up. Oh, and the little shit with the Benson and Hedges and I wasn't about to ask him a second time.

I pushed the penny up onto the flat rim of the ashtray, and then knocked it in a few times to pass some idle moments. I stared at the coin that was now perched over-hanging the hollow of the ashtray. For know particular reason I blew into the ashtray causing an up-draft. This in turn knocked my metal missile onto the bar. I was chuffed to bits, silly sod! All I had to do now was blow harder, concentrating my breath to a smaller area.

Digressing back to my childhood for a moment, I always liked to know the 'ins and out's' of a ducks arse. Never happy just playing with a toy, I wanted to find out how it worked, my Dad was the same. I was given an Etch-a-Sketch on my eleventh birthday, I still have it today. I did the usual squiggles that everybody did, but I couldn't draw a perfect circle. So one afternoon I sat in my bedroom and painstakingly drew lines from one side of the screen to the other. This process removed all of the graphite from the inside and left the internal workings visible.

You will have to forgive me. I have now strayed into the areas of probabilities, percentages and an area called, what's the chance of that happening first time round. Bear with me; it is relevant to this passage. I dropped a tailor-made cigarette out of my mouth whilst at work. I watched as it fell onto the floor and landed on its side. It then bounced back up in an upright position standing on its filter. I was amazed at what I had just witnessed. Come to think of it, I have always liked the thought of long odds. Mainly because of the possibility that it will come off, it must eventually. For example, if you spin a coin a given number of times, say 250,000 times, you must be guaranteed an even amount of heads and tails. But my interest would lie with the probability that at some point the coin would land on its edge. Back to my glass coconut shy.

I lined my launch pad up with the target area, which was three and a half feet up from the bar and approximately seven feet from where I was sitting. I leaned over the ashtray and gave one almighty exhalation of breath. The penny shot high into the air and hit one of the glasses. It bounced off another, ricocheting off and hit the mirrored surface behind the stack of glasses. It landed on the shelf with still a few spins left in its momentum before lying down flat. Blinding, I couldn't find a fault with my project, except I failed to smash any of the glasses. Yet again, I had impressed myself, but not the barman. He heard the end result of my experiment but hadn't a clue as to what had taken place. So acting as causally as you can with two wet socks on, I squelched my way back to a seat near the fire, next to a half open window.

The sun had come out and I watched as the traffic ambled by the pub. A man with tie-back hair and a goatee beard had begun to collect the empties off of the tables. As he neared my table he asked me if I would mind leaving the pub. I looked him up and down noticing on his sleeve was a Tai Chi club badge. I just had a gut feeling that he had probably been doing it longer than me. I came to the conclusion that I had outstayed my welcome. Picking up my still sodden moccasins, I beat a slow, calm retreat. Presumably I went straight home, although my mother seems to think I did wonder off somewhere else. Usual story I'm afraid, I can't remember.

I suppose I must have lost two or three hours to my illness, and the side-effects of the medication, during that day. At five o'clock in the evening Dr Gadhvi had come from Claybury to see how I was. As I recall he was doing his best to persuade me to return to the hospital. But I was having none of it. According to Mum I was so defiant that I ripped up all of my case notes, something I have no recollection of. My alto ego was obviously taking no shit at this stage of the game. Dr Gadhvi left saying he would ring at 7.00 p.m. to see if I had changed my mind. In the meantime a social worker was called as back up, so my Mum wasn't left stranded.

My next memory of that night was four hours later. It was dark obviously, and I now had a flat full of people. Seven o'clock had been and gone and it was now 11pm. What had happened to the daylight hours, and who was the tall bloke with the leather satchel crammed full of paper-work?

Mum was busy in the kitchen making tea and periodically popped into the front room to collect the empty mugs. This was getting more bizarre by the moment. My friends faces all had a pensive look about them. I noticed Bill sitting in a corner with tears falling down his cheeks. I said, "What's the problem, I'm fine." I could see their mouths opening and closing but their words failed to reach my hearing receptors. It was as if I were standing in a triple glazed void. I could hear my voice but no one else's.

At about 11.30 I remember saying to everyone assembled, "This is going to be a very long night." I also informed them that I was off to bed. With my intentions set in crystal, I left them to it. My closest friends, Bill and Chris were there, and their wives Seron and Lorraine accompanied them. They had all rallied round to give my mum some much needed support, bless 'em. I don't know how they put up with me. The man with the Gladstone bag turned out to be a social worker. He was busy getting some background information on me. I was obviously ill again and as usual I was the last to know.

In the safety zone, my bedroom, all was beautifully pitch black. My peace and serenity were blighted only by the muffled voices emanating from the front-room. I was tossing and turning in bed wondering what the hell was going on. As before, I came up with a reason for the late night tea party.

Perhaps I was going through the male equivalent of the menopause. Anyway that's the best I could come up with in the time available. I vividly remember forming all manner of strange contortions with my limbs and body. It was as if I was being pushed and pulled about by an invisible force. This is something that has happened to me before, but during the daylight hours. The involuntary movement lasted I suppose twenty minutes or so. I began to feel frightened by this weird, out of my hands, situation and was glad everybody was still there. I heard a knock at my door. "Can I come in," a male voice said, "Yeah," I replied. It was the social worker.

He asked me to get dressed, and for some reason I gave him the thumbs up sign, much to the relief of my friends and mother. It was now 1.00 a.m. on Tuesday morning. I grabbed my clothes, walked out of my flat and straight into a waiting ambulance. Mum was shattered by this time so Bill and Seron kindly drove her to a family friend's house, where she stayed for a few days. Chris came with me in the ambulance and Rainy, as we called her, followed behind in their car. The last thing I remember being said was Chris asking the driver if he could keep the speed down so Rainy could keep up with us. I may have blacked out for a while, I'm not sure.

I vaguely recall flopping about in the stretcher-bed as the ambulance went round corners. In my stupefied state, I thought I was being taken to see Mark, an inmate that I had met the first time I was admitted to Claybury. Well I would get to meet up with him again, only the stay was to be longer than I had anticipated. I was oblivious that Chris was standing behind me when I got out of the ambulance at the entrance of the hospital. He said it was the most tragic sight he had ever seen. I suppose it's not everyday you see a friend admitted to a loony bin. Chris and I had worked together some years back and became close friends very quickly. You know that positive buzz you get when you meet someone for the first time and you click. Our lives seemed to have run in parallel. Second to Bill, Chris was the brother I never had.

As I walked down the all too familiar gloomy corridor, an image which I shall never be able to erase, I called out Mark's name a few times presuming that he would be there to meet me. My next recollection was sitting opposite a man who was reading something from a sheet of paper, while I, on the other hand, was performing a Tai Chi breathing exercise known only to me. I was in fact being read a section paper. This was a standard procedure for a twenty-eight day stint in the 'fun factory'. He could have been reading the Beano for all I knew. I was too far-gone to make sense of anything at that stage.

CHAPTER THREE

<<<< HIGH AS A KITE >>>>

Now, there is a gap here. Well actually it's more of a chasm. This would be your worst nightmare captured on celluloid. My last memories of that night were of an awful black, dreamlike sensation. More tablets or an injection I suspect. The floors and walls seemed to be made of latex. I walked pitifully into a small dormitory, wearing only my underwear and an oversized blue and white striped gown. As I recall this particular scene, I always begin to fill up, fag break I think…

The illness had stripped me of another part of my dignity even though I was by myself. I don't remember leaving the room where I was sectioned, or who relieved me of my clothing. All I needed was a night-cap and a teddy bear and I could have doubled as Andy, bleedin' Pandy. I think I caught a glimpse of Looby Lu in the bed opposite, well at least I knew I was I the right place.

When I was conscious again, I found myself sitting in the day room of N2. A nurse was telling that me a visitor had come to see me. I had appeared to have been relieved of my Andy Pandy suit and was now dressed in what looked like my own clothes. I wished I knew who kept doing that - it was most disconcerting. Was all this part of an elaborate wind up? It was pissing me off no end.

Although I was heavily medicated, through my blurred vision, no doubt a side-effect of the drugs, I could just make out somebody walking towards me and waving. Wouldn't you know it; it was Bill, smiling from ear to ear.

My first and most obvious question to him was, "How long have I been here?" His reply did not compute on first hearing. "Run that by me one more time?" I said in total dismay. He repeated his answer. "For fuck's sake, that's not possible surely?" I felt around my face to discover that I had almost got a fully grown beard. That would explain this I suppose. Bill nodded in agreement. He looked embarrassed, as if it was his fault I was in hospital again.

I chain-smoked for the next hour or so, still coming to terms with the length of time that I had been incarcerated. Bill informed me that it was the hospitals' decision not to allow anybody to see me as I was far too high. I had been unaware of my surroundings to the tune of 408 hours. What my poor Mum must have gone through. I couldn't believe that it had taken that amount of time to get me in a reasonably coherent state again. Bill left saying he would visit me again soon. I sat in a state of confusion for quite sometime, trying without success to piece back together the last 17 days of my life. Who washed and dressed me? Where did I sleep, did someone have to feed me? Ninety-nine point nine percent of those two and a half weeks is still a blank today. What I can remember I can't even bear to put down on paper.

Weeks later I began to experience flashbacks, or subliminal cuts if you like. The nurses backed up what I had remembered but no more. They said if it's locked away in my subconscious it's probably best left there. I do recall lying down outside the ward office in my coat with my packed bag, telling the staff that I'd had enough of this place and I was off home. Apparently I did this on numerous occasions. I was in fact a fag papers' width away from being put in the 24 lock up ward, N1. Believe me it was not the best accommodation in Claybury Towers! I had taken a liking to setting off the fire alarms on my ward. Well, it broke up the boredom of hospital life no end. I suppose to my mind I thought they were pumping me full of chemicals I knew nothing about; perhaps this was my way of getting them to tell me what they were. Even when I was able to converse with them I never truly understood the full facts surrounding my anti-psychotic medication.

What most people don't realise is that some of these drugs can bring down a charging bull elephant on heat in a matter of minutes. Then the patient has to run the gauntlet of the side-effects, which can be a long, arduous, and sometimes painful journey. If my description so far of hospital life is scaring you, and you thought it couldn't get any worse, it does. N1 was really bad news.

I visited someone who had been placed in there from our ward. Basically it was a medium risk prison area. It had a two-door entry system, and each door was locked behind you as you entered the ward. The dormitory slept eighteen patients. The first thing that struck me was the how tense the atmosphere was. It was as if you were waiting for a riot to go off and so were the staff. All the windows had bars on them. Every item of furniture was secured to the floor. Even the ashtrays were screwed to the tables. The television was encased and set into a wall, with a Perspex protective screen in front of it. Our ward inmate told me that the toilet seats had been removed to prevent them being ripped off and used as weapons.

As with all of the other wards, cigarettes were used as currency. In smokers' terms I was a millionaire and always had a constant supply. On N1 you were only allowed one cigarette an hour. If you had been a naughty boy though, the goal posts were moved slightly and your ration was reduced to one every two hours. In more serious cases your supply was withdrawn altogether. So if you were a nicotine addict, as ninety-five per cent of us were, the nursing staff had you by the nuts. It was a very effective means of control. I was only in N1 for about 20 minutes or so and was glad when we left the 20 by 20 sin bin they called the day room.

It was my next escapade that very nearly put me in the black hole of Calcutta, as I affectionately called it. This was shortly after I purloined a set of ward keys. I was desperate for some decent conversation so I made my way to the ward office and asked the duty nurse if was okay to go in for a chat. Looking around the small room I noticed a big bunch of keys resting in the soap well of the sink in the corner. I asked if I could get myself a drink of water. While the nurse was busy on the phone I picked them up, put them in my pocket and covered them over with my hanky. I made an excuse to leave and headed straight for the locked ward door.

I managed to open it without any problem, and legged it down the stairs to a period of brief freedom. I strolled down the now silent corridor, and headed towards the reception area. I slipped out of the main doors unchallenged, dead chuffed with myself. I threw the keys into a mass of bushes in the grounds and proceeded to walk down the half-mile road that led to the main gates and civilisation.

Opposite the entrance to Claybury was a site to behold, a pub. I sauntered into the car park to find a black cab with the drivers' door slightly ajar. I couldn't resist climbing in and fiddling about with the instrumentation on the dashboard. After a few minutes of mindless touching, pressing and pushing I got out and walked hesitantly towards the pub door. I touched the pubs' brickwork to make sure it wasn't a mirage and I wasn't hallucinating, no, it was rock solid. I felt like a kid that had been let loose in a chocolate factory.

It must have been near closing time now, because I could see the bar-staff cleaning up. Undeterred by this I went into my oasis and ordered a pint of Guinness. As the barman placed it on the bar I said, "Could I owe you for that, only I haven't got any wedge on me at the moment." By the look on the bar steward's face I could see he was none too pleased. As quickly as he poured it out, the accommodating sod chucked the pint down the sink. Six weeks without a beer had made tetchy. Gutted by his unfriendly nature, I decided to stir things up in the car park.

I spied a brand new 4x4 Landrover and thought I would test out its suspension. For a short time I jumped up and down on the running boards on the drivers' side. This felt a bit tame after a while, so I climbed onto the roof via a small ladder on the back of the vehicle and had a proper bounce about. This was much more aesthetically pleasing. At this point of the proceedings, a gin sodden old bint stuck her head out of an upstairs window. Her opening gambit was most unbecoming of a lady, and in true fishwife style she hurled a volley of abuse at me. I must have answered her back but for the life of me I can't remember what I said, more's the pity. I presumed that this ravishing, Gordon's blue-eyed beauty queen, 1947-1987, was the landlord's wife, poor bugger.

She had a face like a clear plastic bag full of crushed walnuts which had been ravaged by time and alcohol. I was soon joined in the car park by the publican and his young son, to the shriek of, "Look Bert, he's climbing all over our new Motor", spoken in a heavy cockney accent. I thought he was going to ask me in for a night-cap. But no, instead he was offering to rip off both of my arms and beat me to death with them. Some people just can't see the funny side of things! Somebody must have phoned the hospital because a Ford Transit van pulled up and out stepped four familiar faces from N2's night-staff.

I was 'helped' into the van and returned to the ward. I tried to do a runner from the main corridor but the nurses were all over me like a rash. I was asked the whereabouts of the ward keys, and I told them roughly where I had aimed them. The trouble was there were literally thousands of bushes in the grounds of the hospital. I told them they had more chance of setting up a threesome with a couple of novice nuns than retrieving the lost keys, but they would insist we searched for them.

So off we trotted into the night with a couple of torches and hope in our hearts! After 20 minutes of fruitless scavenging through the undergrowth the search was abandoned. I was frog-marched back to a single bed side-room on my ward, restrained and injected. As before, I was uninformed as to the contents of the bonus medication. Which I think, looking back, was bloody disgraceful.

I recall turning over on the bed and shouting at one of the nurses, "Why am I here." "You're ill again," came the short reply, "try and get some sleep Neil." A few moments later I passed out. My drug-induced slumber was broken by a burning sensation on my forehead, coupled with a loud banging noise. All of a sudden, the door burst open and in stormed the cleaner from hell. I parted my eye-lids, only to be blinded by a stream of ultra violet light gushing through my window.

The cleaner managed to hit every bit of woodwork in the room. Afterwards, she then proceeded to clout every leg on my bed with her industrial vacuum just for good measure. My ears were overly sensitive at the time and this wasn't the best way to wake me up. I pulled a pillow over my face to mute the row that had invaded my cell of seclusion. Thankfully all went quiet, and my door was closed again. In my solitude, as before, I was left to put my puzzle back together. Thanks to the powerful medication, this was impossible. This was not the first time my short-term memory had been affected.

For the next three days I sat in a vegetative state with an inane grin on my face. By the fourth day I was in a terrible state. I could only walk in short pigeon-steps and my knees were frozen in a half-bent position. Try as I might, I couldn't stand up straight. This predicament left me about eight inches shorter than normal. If that wasn't bad enough, my forearms stuck out in front of me like those of a retired compositor. This part goes from bad to worse. My fingers and thumbs were all pointing towards the floor and like my knees were frozen too. To top it all, every time I went to sit down, literally two seconds later I had to stand up. This compulsion was uncontrollable. The confusion led to tears, lots of them and I was also in a great deal of pain. Bill was the only person to see me like this from the outside world. He said that I looked like ET with a beard. A week later I was still in the same condition.

Nobody appeared to be doing anything to help me. I couldn't sleep on my back or my front, in the end I slept on alternate sides. I would wake up, on the hour, every hour. My spine was the worst affected area. It felt as if the River Dance troop had been practising on it for a month. Eventually, after three weeks of agony and broken sleep, I summoned up the courage to speak to somebody, anybody who would be likely to help me. John Slevin was the man in charge of the ward's medication. I asked him what was wrong with me, and how long I would be stuck like this. He explained.

"You have had a serious reaction to the injection you were given. It's an acute side-effect called, akathisia." He spent well over thirty minutes explaining what I could expect from this debilitating side-effect. The recovery time was open ended, anything from 0 to 14 weeks. I was given an extra tablet to take with my usual medication to help the crippling effects of the akathisia. John added that all forms of medication have side-effects attached to them, even aspirin, but obviously some are more noticeable than others. He wasn't kidding. Of course what I hadn't anticipated was that the so-called anti side-effect tablet had a side-effect all of its own.

Three days later I found out what it was, constipation, wonderful. Not only did I have problems with my external workings, my internal workings were fouled up as well (pun unintended). A week later, I was still having problems sleeping and was given another tablet to take. Guess what, I now had a new side-effect to cope with, blurred vision, mostly with a tad of extra lethargy. If I wasn't walking the corridors or circumnavigating the hospital grounds, in small circles I might add, I could be found propping up a wall in the corner of the day room. You couldn't miss me. I was the blind, bearded, stationary alien with a packet of Ex-lax sticking out of his top pocket!

I'm sure people used me as a coat rack during visiting hours. In the midst of my plight, a fellow inmate leant over my shoulder one afternoon and said in an irritatingly high-pitched voice, "I see you've got it then?" "Got what?" I said indignantly. "You know, it." "Look mate," I said coarsely, "I haven't the faintest idea what you're on about." I was praying for his sake that he wasn't going to say what he said next, but he did, (here it comes), "You know, it!"

My patience had depleted due to the enforced sleep deprivation. I was I think the most agitated I had ever felt. If I wasn't so heavily medicated, I think I might have chinned him. Although having said that, it would have probably been more like a head-butt, bearing in mind I couldn't move my arms. He was really getting on my thrupenny bits and wouldn't leave me alone. As a person not prone to physical violence in any way, shape or form, I'm afraid he encountered the rough edge of my tongue, which in the past had been known to cut a person in half at thirty-six paces! Unfortunately for him I gave him both barrels. I cocked the triggers and fired.

"Listen you berk, either tell me what the fuck you're on about in plain English or fuck off altogether." My 12 bore shots, being at point blank range should have taken his head off; instead they went straight over it. "The shuffle," he said, grinning from ear to ear. To add insult to injury the plank was smiling at me now, oh Jesus. "The Claybury Shuffle." "WHAT?" I replied in disbelief and a raised tone. "The shuffle, the sit down get up syndrome, you've, got... it." Finally it made sense, Christ it took him long enough. I had to smile to myself later on when I had calmed down. He was, of course, right.

In the coming twelve weeks, I completely wore out a brand new pair of trainers. Mile after mile I shuffled, trudging around the hospital corridors and the surrounding woodlands, I couldn't stop myself. As the days passed by, I hoped that all the extra exercise I was doing would bring my symptoms to an end but it didn't. Akathisia would have been a real boon to any war effort. It could immobilise an entire army without a shot being fired. Now there's a thought for world peace!

I got the full use of my legs back after exactly twenty-eight days, and the compulsive shuffling stage was over too.

Two weeks later, I could put my arms down by my side again although not behind my back. After forty-two days of agony I spoke to John Slevin again, still asking the same question. How much longer would I have to put up with this debilitation and pain? "Because you were so incredibly high when you came into hospital I had to slow down your adrenaline rate. What I'm doing now is bringing it back up slowly, so you don't go over the top again." Physio was the next step, hours of it, just to get my joints moving again.

In these sessions the therapist got a group of us to stand in a circle. Then she placed a huge elastic band behind our backs. All we had to do was hold on to it and move in and out. It looked and sounds ridiculously childish, but it stretched our muscles and joints more than they had been in the past weeks. It was difficult to keep a straight face while we were twanging our way round the therapy room, but at least it took our minds off the pain we were all in.

Next on the list of therapy was in the art room, believe it or not. I couldn't see the sense behind it at first. I still couldn't sit down for more than a few seconds, which was adding to my frustration. Can you imagine trying to eat a meal? Now I was expected to paint a picture. I couldn't paint anything when I was at school, my saving grace was that I could design things, and I still have a good eye for colour. Once the barrier of the feeling stupid stage was broken down, and with the help of the occupational therapist, Christine, I felt better about the whole situation. Chris explained she wasn't expecting a Constable or a Renoir, her job was to encourage people to express themselves, which she did.

After each painting or drawing, she would sit and discuss the piece with the patient. It wasn't just a case of bunging a bunch of mentally-challenged people in a room and letting them get on with it. There was so much more to it than that. I did however draw the line at pottery classes, as everything I tried to make ended up looking like an ashtray! In the end I did all my ham fisted, childlike daubing standing up.

The art room was a great relief from the noise of my ward and the rest of the hospital. Second to the relaxation room, it was my favourite place to be. It was always peaceful and calming. Chris was very hot on ambience, and she would only tolerate a certain amount of background noise. The room itself backed on to a huge grassed quadrangle, and it was nice to drift out there for a smoke and feel the sun on my back. It was a welcome respite from the multitude of mental disorder. There were racks of paper and paint everywhere, and pictures on every wall. It reminded me of an oversized version of my art room as a child in the infants' school. There were some brilliant artists there. I particularly liked the pencil drawings. Some days it was as if the creativity was infectious.

People painted their nightmare and dream sequences. Once these pictures of mental torment were out of their mind and down on paper, you could see the genuine relief on their faces. I made a picture of a brightly coloured butterfly from daubs of blue, red and yellow paint. More by luck than judgement, I hasten to add. I folded a piece of cartridge paper in half and aimed the paint on one half. Then I closed the dry half onto the wet side and smoothed it down with my hand so that the colours merged together. When I opened it up the result was a beautiful array of colour. Like me it was a one off, I wished I had kept it now.

My progress towards sitting, walking and general mobility was excruciatingly slow. If the distance to cover was 'the whole nine yards,' I was only proceeding at the rate of a quarter of an inch a day. Frustrating doesn't even come close to describing what I had to contend with. The painting did help; I have no doubt about that. Using a brush aided the manipulation of my finger muscles. Like the art room, the room used for the relaxation group was blissfully serene. On a good day you could have heard a gnat fart! We would lie down on floor mats, close our eyes and listen to Christine's voice. Other than that the only sounds we could hear were, the odd twittering of the birds and the light jangling of some obscure music playing on the cassette player.

The only drawback was that, after thirty minutes in the chill-out department, you had to return to the bedlam of the ward. Still in a trance-like state I would make my way down the winding corridors back to N2. Lunch-time was at 12.30. Unfortunately this was when the relaxation sessions ended. It was poor timing. Everybody who was in the hospital at that time was on the move. The noise was deafening, and it was a rude awakening after such a tranquil half an hour. The other hurdle to cope with was the constant din on my ward, where people argued, fought, or tried to escape.

I had numerous blood tests, never really knowing why or finding out the results. Perhaps they are on my medical records? On a particularly quiet morning, a tall suited man began asking certain patients, including myself, if we would like to take part in some experiments. What would you have said? Call me Mr Picky, but my first thought was bollocks to that. On hearing it meant having extra blood tests, I went with my original thought and declined his kind offer of extra visits to the path lab.

On my second stay in 'happy valley' the life inside and the people within were easier to accept mentally. Sadly there were still some patients on my ward who I recognised from when I was first admitted in February 1993. There was a hierarchy that always sat at the bay window end of the day-room. I only felt comfortable when I had broken the ice with these long-term inmates. Mark was one of these long-stay patients that remembered me when I was brought in for the second time. He helped me to fill in some of the blank spaces, while I was sparked out for the first seventeen days.

CHAPTER FOUR

<<<< MARK, THE INMATES AND THE CLAYBURY SHUFFLE >>>>

On first glance I thought he looked like a psychopath who had been badly photographed by the tabloids, you know, scruffed up to look worse than he actually was. His external appearance put him in the evil son-of-bitch section, but once I got to know him my views changed. After all he had one of the worst mental illnesses I think anyone could have, he was, and still is a paranoid schizophrenic. Mark had a slight frame for his height. He had short, spiky, jet-black hair and a pair of piercing blue deep-set eyes. His teeth were in a bad condition and were heavily stained by hand-rolled tobacco. Like many of us in Claybury, personal hygiene was last on the list of priorities. Mark was one of life's unfortunates and our upbringing couldn't have been more different. One Sunday afternoon, the worst day in any psychiatric hospital save a bank holiday or Christmas Day, he told me about his childhood. Sit back and when you have read this next passage count your blessings.

Mark's father wasn't around the family home much, but when he was everybody suffered. From what I gathered his father was a heavy drinker, and became abusive when he was tanked up. He used to take out all of his insecurities on anybody who was in the house at the time. This was mostly Mark as his mother worked during the day. He was both mentally and physically abused by his alcoholic father and in the end was rejected by his mother. He would bunk off school and was constantly in trouble with the police. At the tender age of 14 Mark was diagnosed with schizophrenia. As a result of being abandoned by both parents, he took drugs and drank alcohol. When this failed to get the much-needed attention he was craving, he turned to something a little more drastic: self mutilation.

I saw the scars he had on both of his arms and wrists. All made with a rusty Stanley knife, he informed me. Mark gave me a lesson in suicide for the uninitiated. "You don't cut across yer wrist if yer seriously finking about topping yerself," he said. Of course I had to ask the question, why? He replied in his usual matter of fact way, "Coz it's 'arder to stitch a vein that's been cut lengff ways." "Hmm, nice touch," I replied morbidly.

The scars on his forearms were massive. The dozen wounds were all over eight inches in length, with five or six one-inch cross-stitches. They looked as though a blind nurse using a blunt size eight knitting needle had sown them up. In the years ahead, Mark's father disappeared off the scene, leaving his mother to cope with their son and his illness. Already emotionally, mentally and physically scarred, Mark couldn't be trusted to take his medication. He either forgot to take it or didn't bother.

Under the rules of his section paper this allowed a doctor to visit Mark at home to inject him once a fortnight. This made sure his medication was in his system, rather than in the dustbin or down the toilet. Once he was administered with his quota of drugs, he was visibly stupefied for a couple of days. He couldn't stay out in direct sunlight for more than a few minutes. If he did his skin became blotchy. This was just one of the side-effects of his potent liquid cosh. However, Mark still managed to retain his wicked sense of humour. I think that's why we clicked when we first met. He had feelings like any other human being, and like me he needed a good laugh. Not that there was much to smile about in Claybury. Mark may have not have looked like it, but he was a kind, polite person underneath his rough looking exterior. He went on to tell me about his failed suicide attempts and how he became a long-stay patient. He had me in fits of manic laughter. His own laugh was contagious. I had to keep asking him to stop so I could get my breath back. One of his most elaborate suicide bids was set in a tube station. The odds of his survival I rated at about one in a million. Mark decided to take a dive under some 1967 rolling stock.

My first bout of uncontrollable giggling began when he told me he bought a return ticket! He stood right next to the tunnel where the tube entered the platform. Mark made his lunge but mis-timed the speed of the train. Instead of ending up under the wheels and a quick death, he landed head first between the first two carriages. The train carried him in this position down the whole length of the platform. When it came to an abrupt halt it dropped him straight into an inspection pit. To add insult to very little injury, no one saw what had happened. He dusted himself off and made a swift exit from the station. Marks next venture landed him up in front of the beak, facing an eight year stretch in one of her Majesty's hotels. However, because of his illness, he was granted a reduced sentence if he agreed to go into a mental institution, what a choice! He plumped for the 'happy factory,' which knocked three years off his penance to society.

Still intent on gaining some attention, he went out one morning with a loose idea of holding up his local sub-post office. His choice of weapon, a sawn-off cucumber wrapped in a black bin liner! At this point I had another laughing fit. What made it worse Mark told me that he had queued up. To this day I still have a vivid mental picture of this scene, and grin when I recount this story. Mark was next in line, concealed cucumber at the ready. He asked the cashier to fill up his carrier bag with money. The bloke behind the counter looked bemused until Mark unzipped his jacket and brandished the first two inches of his twelve-bore salad fruit. With no cash forthcoming, Mark tried again to get his message across. "Look you dozy bastard," he said losing his rag. "Fill up the bag or I'll blow yer fuckin' 'ead off." Before the teller had time to panic, the customer behind Mark came to the rescue. He had overheard the hold-up demands and, before Mark knew it, he was lying face down on the post office floor. The public-spirited man was now sitting on Mark's back, forcing his hands up towards his neck. Well, at this stage of the story I was in need of a cylinder of oxygen. My lungs felt as though my intestines were throttling them. I waved at him to stop talking as I felt my chest cavity begin to implode. He was no better, we only had to make eye contact and the whole manic giggling fit started again. I laughed so much that I couldn't smoke for half an hour afterwards. What Mark didn't know of course was the bloke standing behind him in the queue was an off-duty police officer. Now what are the chances of that happening?

This semi quiet Sunday of jollity was blighted by the sound of a new arrival to N2, Malcolm. He was a tall, thin, balding chap wearing thick black-rimmed glasses. From a distance he appeared to be dressed in a matching 'Bacofoil' two-piece number. As the policeman helped Malcolm into the day room, I could see it was a silver thermal suit. My initial thought was that he had taken a dive in a local river to end it all? I never did find out. Mark recognised Malcolm, and said in his usual dulcet tones, "Ere' he comes, all right Malc." Then at the top of his vocal range he shouted, "Houston we have a problem, the Martians have landed in Claybury." I creased up. Even the copper had a smile on his face. As I was about to find out, Malcolm was a compulsive talker when he became ill. He didn't draw breath from one sentence to the next. He sat down next to Mark and I at the bay window end of the day room. After a short burst of verbal drivel, Mark in his inimitable style said, "Fer fuck sake Malc, shut up will yer." We then had to listen to and endless stream of apologies. "Sorry," He kept saying, repeating it over and over again. "I try to stop talking but I can't, I annoy everybody in the end." He wasn't kidding. "Sorry, see, there I go again. Sorry, ah sorry, sorry." Mark repeated his plea for silence. Malcolm managed to keep 'schtum' for fifteen seconds but that was all. He was literally biting his bottom lip. Suddenly he burst forth with a torrent of unrelated spiel. He couldn't keep his mouth shut for love nor money, poor bloke. Mark and I made a hasty retreat to the tearoom, leaving Malcolm in his own world to a two-way conversation by himself.

Most of the patients were easy to get on with, but then we were all on pretty hefty drugs. I would like to think that we weren't over-prescribed with drugs. The thought did cross my mind on more than one occasion, especially as I saw so many people walking around like zombies. In that soporific state you are powerless and easily controllable, not forgetting vulnerable too. There were however two 'oiks' on my ward that everybody did their best to avoid. The first was a young black man. I'm not xenophobic by any means but this bloke really took the biscuit. He had a real hatred of white women during his illness. He seemed quite a well-balanced bloke to me as he had a chip on both shoulders! He never missed a chance to verbally abuse the ladies whenever he could. This was usually done in the line-up at 'tablet time' which was four times a day in most cases, or when we queued for our meals. The staff certainly had their hands full when he was on the prowl. He would get hold of drink or cannabis, which was freely available if you moved in the right circles. Unfortunately, these drugs counter-acted his medication. His daily routine revolved around sitting in various corners of the ward, hissing at people like a pissed off rattlesnake.

Another patient on the ward who was a pain in the arse was a bloke I nicknamed 'the weasel,' among others. He was a horrible little shit who thought the ward revolved around him. As far as I could work out, he was in for detoxification but, like the first bloke I mentioned, he also managed to get hold of alcohol and weed. I was still in a weak condition when we first set eyes on each other. I couldn't have told you what time of day it was, come to that I couldn't have told you what day it was either.

I remember a group of us were sitting in the day room. It must have been a ward round or something. I had run out of cigarettes, which was unusual for me. Sitting opposite me was the dreaded 'weasel.' He got up and made his way to the tea trolley. As he did so I noticed a packet of Benson & Hedges lying at the back of his chair. It hadn't occurred to me that they belonged to him. I opened the box, stuck one behind my ear and lit a second one, putting the packet back where I found it. Puffing away to my heart's content I slid into the toilets thinking I had got away with my day-light pilfering. When I returned to my seat smoking the second cigarette the gold pack was still there. It was almost shouting at me to pick it up and slip it in my pocket. The cigarette box shone like a beacon as the sun's rays hit it. The temptation was too great to ignore. I headed towards the toilets again to check the bounty.

Unbeknown to me 'stoat face' must have been watching my every move. As quickly as the bog door shut behind me it opened again. He shouted, "Oi, you seen my snout pal?" Quick to have a smart put-down, I was going to say, "Yes, it's between your gob and your eyes, all you're missing is a set of whiskers." But he looked incensed, as if he had seen the 'red haze' and his eyes looked like a couple of ordinance survey maps, so I thought better of it. Pity though, if I do say so myself it was a blinding line to fire back at him, particularly considering how drugged up I was at the time. We were now retina to retina as I handed over the hospital currency back to him. I could tell he wasn't too impressed with the amount of cigarettes that were missing. In the friendliest way he knew how the wiry little wretch told me, if I touched them again he would punch my lights out. Not being one given to violence I gave him a wide berth after that.

On the odd occasion 'rat fink' had visitors, I had a chance to work out what sort of background he had come from and how he was dragged up. True to form I wasn't disappointed by my findings. His dad and step-trollop were the most frequent visitors and what a win double they turned out to be. The father was a tall, over-weight, over-bearing bigot covered in naff looking tattoos. To add to this adornment, he was wearing far too much Argos gold. His vocabulary comprised of an expletive every other word and he had the IQ of a radiator. His peroxide bint reeked of Halfords' top-selling perfume. I was in two minds as to which one it was, 'Hint of Gusset' or 'Eau de Brothel.' She too was dripping in an over-abundance of catalogue gold, and her brain capacity was equalled with pond life. In the unlikely event they were selected for Mastermind, their chosen subjects might have been, alcohol, 1945 onwards, and swearing through the ages.

They seemed to think that there wasn't much wrong with their little Hitler, well nothing that a good clump wouldn't sort out. To help him through his detox step-mater and pater took the little shit to the pub for the afternoon session. Some people defy belief. If he's not dead from alcoholic poisoning or drug abuse, I imagine he is still on the outside causing havoc wherever he goes.

After eight weeks I was seen fit to be included in the ward round. This consisted of hanging around the day room for hours on end, waiting to be seen by the head shrink. Ward rounds were daunting. I felt as if I was going up in front of a parole board, which I suppose I was in a way. Along with Dr Gadhvi sat a social worker, the head nurse and, more often than not, a trainee. The purpose of these meetings was to ascertain the individual progress of the patients. Depending on their findings you began a build up towards weekend leave. This began with a couple of hours away from the confines of the hospital. It was difficult to see any improvement in myself, even after my discharge from the hospital. All I seemed to do was chain smoke through the terminal boredom of each day. The days were painfully long. Eventually the time came for my two-hour respite in the outside world. I couldn't see the need to acclimatise myself to being away from the hospital. Unfortunately I was totally unaware that I had become institutionalised in a relatively short period of time. I was also forgetting I was now a full-blown care in the community statistic.

I was champing at the bit to get away from hospital environment. The lighting, the rooms, the food, the people and the infernal noise were all getting on my tits. I was asked how I was coping with my debilitating akathisia. Ten weeks after the injection to calm me down, my fingers were still painfully swollen. I still couldn't put my arms behind my back, even after that amount of time, and my spine still ached like hell. Every vertebra felt bruised to the core. The most frustrating part of the whole episode was not being able to sit down for more than a few moments at a time. My involuntary movements, coupled with the agonising pain, would have tested the patience of a saint. The nurse's main concern was that if I couldn't sit still for too long how would I cope with being enclosed in the confines of a car? The compulsion to get up once I had sat down was uncontrollable. It was as if my hips had strings on them. Every time I went to park my butt down, invisible puppeteers made me stand up. It was funny at first, but after weeks and weeks of this it became bloody irritating. It was decided that if by the following Saturday I could keep my bum on a seat for at least ten minutes, I would be allowed to go out for a couple hours.

The next four days dragged of course. Waiting, that's all we ever seemed to do as patients. With the thought of two whole hours away from all these ill people, which after a while begins to drag you down, I had become obsessed with trying to keep my bottom on a chair. The only way I could sit in near comfort was to turn a chair around so the back faced my stomach. Even so I was still in a great deal of pain. The fateful day arrived. I had to admit to Trisha that I couldn't sit still for the ten minute period suggested. I was nearly in tears.

"How long can you manage then?" She asked. "About seven minutes, it's not long enough is it?" I replied. "Do you still want to go out for the afternoon?" "More than anything," I replied, "just to get away from this place." "Okay listen," she said smiling, "it's a positive sign your on the mend but we must make sure Bill is aware how serious your condition is, go and give him a call." Those words were a shot in the arm to me. I was buzzing all the way down to the pay phone. I felt like a kid going out on his first school trip. It was an unbelievable sensation of happiness.

As promised, Bill turned up on the dot of 12 o'clock and the staff briefed him about the implications of suffering from akathisia. As I sat in the confinement of Bill's passenger seat, the compulsion to stand up overwhelmed me. Bill, as patient as ever, said, "Don't worry, take your time, there's no rush mate." We sat and had a smoke, idly chatting about this and that as we looked over the grounds of the hospital. It was a cloudless, blue sky day. The sun was just behind us casting long shadows from the tall fir trees that lined the car park. "Fit?" Bill said. "Yep," I replied. "C'mon then, lets get you away from this place for a while."

We headed down the long approach towards the main gates and out into the main road. I felt odd, as if I were retracing a bad dream. My world was on hold again, so why wasn't everybody else's? My overriding fear was realising that I had to catch up with the rest of the planet again. In the bombproof environment of a psychiatric hospital, this is something you forget very quickly. As the car neared the first set of traffic lights I began to panic. I said to Bill, "I'm in trouble here mate; I've got to get out." As the words left my lips, the lights changed to green and the urge subsided. I was fine as long as the car was moving, but the slightest hint that we were going to slow down or, even worse, stop, I began to rock back and forth in my seat.

As we got closer to home I looked in complete awe at the shops and people that I recognised walking up or down, as the case may be, in Station Road. It seemed such a long time since I had walked up there by myself. I was in a state of shock. As we drove around all the roads I had known since I was five years old, I began to feel out of place. Although I didn't say anything to Bill at the time, I was beginning to think I should have stayed where I was. The very place I was so desperate to get away from suddenly had a strange appeal.

I felt deeply ashamed of myself and embarrassed of my appearance. So much so that I spent the first 15 minutes apologising to Bill's wife, Seron, for the state I was in. I had a full beard, I couldn't sit still and I had lost over a stone in weight. I would have looked more at home in an Oxford Street doorway rather than in Bill and Seron's clean, suburban home. I couldn't even remember when I had last bathed properly. To add to this glorious feeling of well being I was medicated up to my eyebrows. In the end Bill said, "Stop worrying about what you look like, park your self somewhere, you're among friends." Then he handed me a cup of tea.

It was such an odd feeling being back in familiar territory. As I walked into their back room I looked and touched most of their ornaments and pictures before trying to sit down. I didn't want to wake up in a hospital bed to find a crowd of people standing over me. To this day I don't like lots of people standing near me. Convinced I was in reality, I sat for as long as my brain would let me.

Questions began forming a queue in my head as I sat sipping my tea in silence. All my emotions surfaced at once and I was thrown into a fit of confusion. Why was I in hospital? What was wrong with me? Then the pace of my questioning picked up. Did I have a job? What did I do for a living? The flat, the flat, if I've got a mortgage who is paying that? Who's putting electric on the key? I was calm for one moment and paranoid the next. I laughed at a whimsical thought that had crossed my mind then a millisecond later I was in tears. I think it was at that point that I realised just how long I had been out of circulation. Bill put his arm around me and said, "It's all right, you have had a serious break-down but you will get over it in time." Later on we sat down for lunch or rather they did. I had to stand up for most of mine. My back was giving me so much grief. "Why don't try sitting down at the table?" Bill inquired. "I wish I could mate." "You're such a tart Walton," he replied sarcastically. So for the last five minutes of the meal I reverted to turning the chair round, resting my forearms on the back rest. At the time I couldn't fully describe to my hosts just how much pain I was in. So, apart from the River Dance troop that had been practising on my spine, I will endeavour to explain the agony to you. Bear in mind that I was in pain everyday for three months, here goes.

Imagine an operation where you have had your spine removed. Each vertebra has been hit several times with a claw hammer, and then crudely rasped with a half round bastard file. It gets a little worse from this point onwards. Every alternate vertebrae had now been turned round a full 180 degrees and then banged back into position by an irate eight year old with a croquet mallet. It's still not over yet. Any remaining lubricant has been removed by an industrial suction pump. That's about it, oh I forgot to mention, and when your spinal column is replaced it is put back the wrong way up.

After ham-fistedly eating my meal I went and sat in the front room and relaxed with a filter coffee. I had forgotten what good food tasted like. I shouldn't complain, I know, but I'm sure one of the hospital concoctions was donkey stew! This might sound like a rash statement, but when I was first admitted to Claybury with clinical depression I heard, or thought I heard, the braying of a donkey. I said nothing and waited to see if Bill clocked the same noise. Over a cup of tea I heard the braying again, only it was much louder this time. I looked at Bill and he looked at me and he said, "I wonder if he's on your ward?" As we peered through one of the windows in the tearoom I saw two donkeys stroll past. The hospital had a small sanctuary with in the grounds. What worried me the most was one of them had a leg missing. I replied, "I hope not, unless it is a new form of therapy, it looks like they are eating him a bit at a time!"

Without realising it I had managed to remain seated for more than twenty minutes. Bill called from the kitchen, "Can I get sir anything else, peel you a grape maybe?" "No, one's quite replete thanks, although you could get the butler to run the iron over the FT for me!" A little later on in the day I remembered there were two things I desperately needed. They were basic requests but at the time they were of paramount importance to me. "Do us a favour Bill," I said, "sorry to be a pain in the arse but you couldn't shave this shit of my face could you, it's driving me nuts?" My final demand was the use of Bill and Seron's bathroom. "I must stink like a polecat," I said. "I wondered where the pong was coming from," he retorted.

I felt so desperately frail and beholden, and it is this very scenario that devours a depressed person's confidence.

Bill began to clip away at my facial growth. Once he had cut off all he could with the scissors, he shaved off the remaining fuzz with his razor. What a gorgeous feeling it was to be clean-shaven again. I still felt dirty though. This made me wonder how or who washed me during my seventeen day blackout? I don't know if I was approachable or not. Looking at some of other patients in varying degrees of their fluctuating illnesses, sad to say I think I was probably left to my own devices.

Bill shouted down to me from upstairs and informed that my second favour was in progress. I couldn't wait. I managed to wash my hair, face, arms, legs and stomach but had to ask Bill if he could wash my back for me, I did feel a prat. I had forgotten my shoulder joints weren't fully functional and washing my own back was still out of my grasp. I leant forward and Bill, bless him, massaged the soap into my aching back. It felt wonderful. "I'll give you a month to stop that," I said to him, "how much will the 'extras' cost me sweetie?" "I'll give you the bill before you leave big boy." "Before I knock-off for the day sir," Bill said with his tongue stuck firmly in his cheek, "would you like me to digest your meal for you; I've done everything else for you so far today?" "Passmore I said, if I had the strength, I'd give you a slap." He grinned at me and left me to languish in the hot, steamy atmosphere of his family bathroom.

As I stood up to get out of the bath I felt dizzy. I think it was a combination of the steamy room and my medication.

I wrapped myself in two large white towels and slid slowly down the tiled wall opposite the bath in a dazed state. The next thing I remember was waking up laying face down on Bill and Seron's bed. I felt a bit awkward when Bill roused me from my cat-nap. The hot bath had loosened all of the bones in my spine. I felt so relaxed that I had trouble keeping my eyes open. The reason I didn't wash, apart from the chronic pain I was in, was because, like the sleeping quarters in Claybury, the bathroom had very little privacy. It was a large, cold room with a huge bath to the left of the door as you went in. On the right hand side were three large sinks with tatty looking mirrors above them. All that separated the sinks from the bath was an enormous green plastic sheet that was suspended from an aluminium rail. On the floor at the side of the bath was an anti-slip mat, one half of which was always immersed in a pool of cold water.

I left it and left it before baring my skin to the uninviting washing facilities, hoping upon all hope that no one would come in while I was trying to wash. I was just about to chisel off my nether garments when the door burst open. In marched one of the nurses doing a body count, wouldn't you Adam and Eve it. "It's me, Neil," I said, "Okay," he replied. As he shut the door behind him it caused a belt of cold air to circulate around the already freezing cold bathroom. As I peered into the bath I found it was littered with toe nail clippings and a mass of pubic hair. Needless to say I emptied the bath and washed away as much human debris before baring my rancid skin to it. I put some of my clothes back on and refilled the tub.

By now I was bloody freezing. Thankfully I managed to get into the bath without being disturbed but it didn't last long. There's nothing worse than when a stranger or two breaks the silence by grunting, burping or farting while you are having a soak. It was a hideous event in one of my many hospital admissions. As with childbirth, all your dignity is lost in one fell swoop but in a psychiatric hospital the effects seem to last a lot longer. I only used the bathroom once in 14 weeks. It repulsed me so much that I would only wash at friends' houses during my away-day trips from the hospital.

I couldn't get over how peaceful Bill's house was. Even with two of his three children present. It was nice to feel the carpet between my toes again. Being in a normal sized room made a change too. Another treat was actually hearing what was being said on the television, something that was impossible to do on the ward. It was both loud and distorted or people would be taking over the dialogue, either way it was bloody annoying. I realised just how therapeutic that first afternoon away from the 'hell hole' was for me. It was a turning point in my recovery; it was the first time that I noticed a difference in myself without it being prompted by somebody in a white coat.

I was just getting used to the peace and quiet when I heard a clock strike five. I would soon have to face the mayhem of the 'fun factory.' I didn't want to go back and I think Bill could sense my feelings. I sat in my chair with my head down, rather like a child would who had just been told off. Trisha, my head ward nurse had said to Bill before we left, if I coped with the afternoon outing I could do the same thing the following weekend. Hearing this bit of news did put a smile back on my face, I must admit, and the ride back was a lot less fraught. I was more relaxed for one thing; even so I couldn't stop myself from rocking back and forth every time Bill's car slowed down or came to a halt. I arrived back on N2, beaming from ear lobe to ear lobe, pointing out to three of the night staff my clean-shaven face. They were all interested to know how my afternoon went. I told them it was okay, but a bit scary at the same time. "I wasn't expecting to feel so nervous." I said. "That's the first and biggest hurdle you've had to face and you've coped really well." "But why was I so frightened?" "Institutionalisation, you're in a vulnerable condition at the moment and it doesn't take long to become reliant on others." She went on, "Some patients can't even bare the thought of leaving the hospital grounds. To them it's a safety zone. You should be pleased with yourself." "Yeah I suppose, I didn't realise just how dependant I had become on you lot," I replied. "Well that's what we are here for Neil; you have a serious illness and we will help you get through it." The conversation tailed off at that point. I said to her, "But nobody can see what I've got, I wish I had two broken legs." She smiled knowingly and said, "We will talk about that side of your illness soon." With that she went back into the ward office to take a phone call.

In my weakened state, I sat at a table near the office and took stock of my weekend achievement. The awful thing was I was actually glad to be back in the confines of the hospital. The people were more like me. It must be the old safety in numbers theory. Not only that, I was in an environment where I didn't have to think for myself, which you can get quite attached to. I was woken at eight in the morning. Breakfast, dinner and an evening meal were laid on for me. Mind you, having said all of that, I couldn't have cooked for myself, not the state I was in. To a degree I felt as though I was being brain-washed back into society, with the aid of a trick cyclist and an endless supply of heavy-duty anti-psychotic drugs.

I did feel like a prize tart when I thought about what had taken place at Bill's house. All I had done was visit a friend at his home, something I had done countless times before I became ill. You wouldn't think a person could be so fragile. You could be built like an ox, and depression will crush you flat. It could be happening to you, a relative or a close friend as you read this passage! Beware the 'slipping clutch' syndrome. If you've never seen a person suffer and recover from a complete nervous break-down, I suggest you look in at your nearest psychiatric hospital. It is a great leveller. I'm of the mind now that the subject of mental illness should be added to the school curriculum; perhaps in the students final two years.

CHAPTER FIVE

<<<< THE FINAL KNOCKINGS >>>>

I was entering my ninth week in the 'sin bin.' My back was still giving me jip, and all of my digits were still badly swollen. It was time to see Jon Slevin again. Even he admitted it was the worst reaction to injected medication he had seen in twenty years. "Let's see," he said as he flicked through my medical notes. "Okay, are you sleeping better now?" "Yeah, I'm getting about five hours in, which is two hours more than I have been getting," I replied. "Hmmm, it's still not enough is it? He said. "I feel ratty all of the time." "Well it's hardly surprising; sleep deprivation can reduce people to tears." "Yeah I know, I've reached that stage now. Not only that, my spine still aches from top to bottom." "What about your arms, how far back can you move them?" "Not far," and I showed him. "Oh dear," he replied, "Your shoulder joints are still badly swollen. I'll give you some stronger pain killers to relieve the pain in your spine and some anti-inflammatory tablets for your shoulders, which should do the trick. You should be clear of all the side-effects within three to four weeks."

My head dropped. "I don't think I can take much more of this Jon, I'm in bloody agony." "Right, okay, first things first, let's treat the pain." He got up and opened the medication room. Jon returned with a tumbler of water and two large white tablets that a horse would have been proud to swallow. "Take these, how long have you been in this amount of pain?" "About six and a half weeks," I replied. "My dear boy why on earth didn't you tell someone?" "I didn't want to be a nuisance," I replied drying my eyes. "Give the tablets twenty minutes or so to get in your system and I'll come and check on you again. Don't ever hesitate to ask for me if you are in any discomfort Neil, that's what I am here for."

The pain subsided and Jon returned to finish off our conversation bless him. "Stick with the relaxation and art sessions, and we will soon have you out of the woods." He was a lovely bloke and his attention to detail within his field of work was immaculate. He had a knack of making you feel as if you were the only patient he was treating. Even the head psychiatrist had to wait in line if Jon was explaining a patient's medication to them. He was always in demand on N2. One of his traits I particularly admired was that he would never leave a patient in the lurch or pass people off to a junior.

During the next four weeks I was to have six trips away from the 'fun palace.' Most were during the day, but to add a little variation I had a few evening excursions. This was the build up to a whole weekend at home in my flat. Mum, as ever, would be on hand as I couldn't use anything mechanical, especially if it had small moving parts. Nearly four and a half months was to pass before I regained the full use of my hands. So cooking, washing and housework were impossible, but funnily enough this condition didn't prevent me from smoking!

My mother, as I am sure you will agree, was without doubt a tower of strength throughout the darkest days of my life. She would travel the thirty-two mile journey to Chingford and stay with her old friends, Myrtle and Reg Woods. Using their house as a base, Mum could visit me during the week and rest at the week-ends. It was a two bus journey from Chingford to my appalling place of confinement. In my dazed condition it was wonderful to see Mum arrive and get off the bus at the stop in the grounds of Claybury. The hardest part was watching as she boarded the bus on the return trip. I still don't know who was more upset when visiting time was over. I said to her on one occasion, "Will they get me better Mum?" meaning the hospital. "Yes of course they will," …with a detectable air of uncertainty in her motherly voice. I felt ridiculous, as I'm sure you can imagine. I was a grown man, and yet I still needed that assurance to make me feel safe and secure.

After seven ward rounds and six afternoon/evenings away from the hospital I was asked if I would like to try a week-end at home. I said yes without thinking, totally oblivious of how cocooned I had become by hospitalisation. In my head things were running at a much slower rate compared to the outside world. My thought process was, and still is, painfully slow, which makes me feel overly self-conscious. I can't concentrate on the smallest of tasks unless am I isolated from any background noise. Just after each high episode, my sense of hearing was so acute I could hear a butterfly fart at thirty-five yards! The thought of two whole days of peace sounded very appealing. No banging, clattering, queuing for meals or medication, and best of all no screaming patients.

My thoughts turned to the things other than the benefits of forty-eight hours of serenity. My bed came top of the list. Oh my bed, my great big comfortable bed, I couldn't wait to slip under the duvet. Not only that, I would have washing facilities all to myself. This was getting better and better, the more I thought about it. The other bonus of course was that there wouldn't be an entourage of fag poncers within a four mile radius. No inane conversations about what life was like inside a ping pong ball and nobody in my face, brilliant. Then came the stark reality of the situation. It crashed over and drenched me from head to toe. It was Mum, a pensioner, and a pathetic version of my old self against the rest of the outside world. Suddenly a forty-eight hour pass didn't sound like such a good idea after all. All I could do, now I was more aware of my surroundings, was boil a kettle and make a cup of tea. That was the sum total of my recuperation and functions after being in a sanatorium for two and a half months. The weekend was only two days away.

My biggest fear now was how I would cope without the hospital's regime to blanket me. I was reassured again and again and again by the ward staff that, if it wasn't working out, I could phone and speak to somebody day or night. If the worst occurred, and panic set in, I could return to the hospital and try again the week-end after. Bill met me in reception at 4 o'clock on Friday as arranged, along with my mother of course. I was in relatively good spirits as we left the grounds of 'happy valley.' As I reclined somewhat awkwardly in Bill's passenger seat the enforced rocking began and lasted the entire journey home. The ride as before was a day dream experience. Once I settled in at home the dreamlike state remained, and I began having flashbacks of the period prior to being coerced back to Claybury. It wasn't the kind of home-coming I was expecting or wanted. It was awful. No one else could see, hear or feel what I was experiencing. Interestingly enough each flashback was unaccompanied by the sense of smell.

As in Bill's home I touched, lifted, moved and replaced most of my household possessions until I was satisfied it was all real. Mum put the kettle on, while I sat in silence waiting for the obligatory cup of tea. As I sipped at my mug, I surveyed my front-room, now feeling strongly out of place in my own surroundings. My mind drifted back to when I was married. I could hear my children running down the hallway and into their bedrooms screaming their little heads off as they went. At that time in my life, Dad was still on the planet and living with Mum at No. 9. I was blissfully employed, having the time of my life at a large printing company called, D.S. Colour International, or 'the nut house', as it came to be known by the people who turned up there each day. I miss that place like a stevedore misses the docks. My sister was married and living in Vienna.

All this had now changed. My marriage had failed, my long standing job ended in redundancy and I was drinking heavily. I gained a new job, only to be made redundant four and a half months later, (two months before Christmas), and then my father died. My wonderful life at that point in time was like the nitrogen dipped poppy that fell off the lab technician's bench. I worked my butt off for twenty-four years, trying to do things the way my Dad did, only to be reduced to an insolvent gibbering wreck.

After this second incarceration, I had lost all sense of where I belonged.

Depression has an open ended incubation period, and it could quite easily remain undetected for years. Then the bastard implodes on its host when they haven't got the physical and, more importantly, the mental strength to fight it. Clinical depression takes no prisoners. I had lost my identity through mental illness, and didn't know myself any more. I felt as if I had been stripped down to my underwear and left on the centre spot just before the final whistle went at the 1966 World Cup. After the media, the players and all of the fans had left the ground, I was left to clear up the mess by myself. My second break-down was a public execution without the death. Normality, what ever that was, or is, had ceased. I now faced the arduous task of having my brain re-set by the powers at be. At the time I couldn't remember what I liked or disliked. My data banks had been wiped clean. Both my long and short term memory were badly affected. All of my natural senses, except my hearing, which made up for loss of all my other senses, were deadened by heavy medication like the dampers on piano wire.

In one particular ward round, I was asked by a trainee nurse how I felt in myself at that precise moment. My reply reduced her to a head down, pen biting, paper shuffling, foot twitching, finger picking nerve bag. I only said 11 words, but they cut her in half like a Samurai sword from head to anus. Slowly and quietly I said to her, "I feel as though a piece of my brain has died." A morgue silence consumed the oxygen in the large room and the six people in front of me. Not even the head shrink could come to her rescue.

I made the tea this time, just to make myself feel useful I think. This was the only household task I could perform unaided. As the kettle began to boil, I immediately thought of the hospital. No matter what department you were in, there was always an area set a side for a brew-up. Like cigarettes, it went with the territory. Half way through my tea I started to feel agitated and said to mum I was going for a walk, I didn't know where, I just had to get out. Ironically I felt claustrophobic in my flat after surviving in the gargantuan living quarters of Claybury Hospital. I still had a tad of the 'Claybury shuffle' with me. At its peak, I was told by a nurse, it was possible for a patient suffering from akathisia to cover three miles a day. The side-effect alone was enough to test the patience of any human being.

As I walked around familiar territory it began to rain. I didn't care. It felt homely somehow, and pleasant on my face. I looked through the windows of the houses I passed, wondering if there was anybody behind the glass suffering as I was. Like my mind in Claybury, the lights were off and everybody was out to lunch!

On my first Saturday of freedom for two months, Judie, my ex-wife was bringing my two beautiful boys to see me. I desperately wanted to see them, but in the same instance I felt scared for myself and for them. I was making the most of being able to lie flat out on my bed, when I heard a knock at the front-door. There was a tap on my bedroom door and mum reinforced the reality of what I imagined to be another drug-induced dream sequence. I opened my eyes and looked up to see two little people, one a little larger than the other, but both bigger than I remembered, amble past my doorway. I felt embarrassed but not in a bad way. About as embarrassed as you would be if a famous personality was stuck in a lift with you, what do you say to them? I opened my arms out wide and hugged their gangly frames.

They were so pleased to see me. It was of course an emotionally charged scene. I choked back as much saline solution as I could, masking my feelings with as much light-hearted banter as I could muster. It must have been a pathetic sight. I listened, absolutely captivated by their squeaky little voices. I remember being unable to resist touching their petite faces. At the time it was hard to believe I was their father, or a father at all come to that. Jack seemed unaffected by my absence, but obviously realised that he had not seen me for quite sometime. He was just seven. How do you explain manic depression to a child of that age? Judie did her best and told the boys that my illness made me feel very, very sad. There really wasn't anything else she could say. I hoped them seeing me made things easier to understand in their little minds.

Daniel went through a spate of lashing out while he was at school. He was so frustrated that he couldn't help me in some way, and it manifested itself in the form of violent outbursts. Once Judie informed his school of my ill heath, it was easier for his teachers to monitor the situation. He was ten at the time. The boys were only with me for an hour, but that was as much as I could cope with. I was emotionally drained long after they had left to go home. I hadn't seen them for approximately ten weeks.

Only once during that week-end did I feel like returning to the safety zone of the hospital. After much deliberation, I manage to overcome my feelings. I decided to make the most of my freedom while I could. I didn't mention it to Mum as she had had enough upheaval already. Mentally at least, I turned a few corners in those two days. But after the routine I had been used to in the 'sin bin,' I could see I was going to have a fight on my hands etching out a new one in the outside world. As I said before I had lost my identity and the luxury of knowing myself. This floundering was to stay with me for well over 12 months after my release from Claybury.

Fourteen weeks after developing the first painful symptoms of akathisia, which had in part crippled me for that entire period; it finally released ninety-eight percent of its grip from my body. On both Saturday and Sunday, I awoke at bang on the dot of eight o'clock. The only thing missing was a herd of nurses trying to get me up and out of bed. I turned on my side, lit a cigarette and luxuriated in the chapel-like silence that my bedroom always had. I didn't feel as if I had done much during the two day break as I recall. In the end it was nice to be in my own surroundings for that brief period. Mum and I walked up to Bill's house, and of course I remember the boys coming to see me, but If I had blinked on Friday afternoon, when Bill came to pick me up, I would have missed the week-end altogether. On the way up to Bill's abode, Mum and I walked past the pub where I did my 'physics project' with the penny and the glass coconut shy. Mum was totally unaware of what had happened in there of course. I, on the other hand, walking in silence just behind her, began having a series of flashbacks of the entire event at a rate of four frames per second, backwards and forwards.

I haven't a clue as to what we ate at Bill and Seron's, or if we stayed for dinner at all. The whole forty-eight hours was a bit of a smudge, if you know what I mean. I know had a great sense of not belonging in my flat, conscious of the fact that in the future it would be repossessed. I knew then that I would never recover in time to catch up with the colossal arrears that I owed my mortgage lender after this second total nervous break-down. That notice was indelibly etched on my frontal lobe for months and months and months. Everyday for two and a half years I waited for the letters to drop on my mat. As well typed and worded as they were, they might just as well have said, "oi wanker, stump up the cash or we'll take your bricks and mortar away!"

I was now financially ruined. The only post I seem to get were bills and those cheery reminders from my lenders, in pristine white envelopes, relating what, to me, was a vast amount of debt. People have committed suicide for less. The worst part was not being able to stop it happening. I recall saying time and again to people, "I wish I could get better faster." It wasn't to be. Everything I had worked for was going to be taken away from me. Mostly due to circumstance, but largely due to mental illness. Adding insult to my mental condition I lost my home and the pension that ran alongside the mortgage. No matter how many people said, "Don't worry", it didn't cut the mustard I'm afraid. Why would it, they weren't technically going to be homeless. It is no surprise to me that people with a mental disorder end up residing in places like cardboard city. Depression is a classless disorder.

Everything that had ever gone wrong in my life happened in that building. I was so sensitive to things at the time I could actually feel the negativity in each room; mostly in the kitchen. I should have gleaned something by our moving date perhaps, the 6/6/86! I am just as sensitive to cold spots in rooms today. Okay you can stop laughing now. My only retort to those who do snigger at me is, I know what I know and that's the end of the conversation! At some point in my life, somewhere I will meet a person who will be able to explain things to me in greater depth. You don't go telling people you've had countless psychic events during your life, even more so after having a break-down. Well not unless you are in responsive company, such as Bill and Seron, who have had their share of psychic experiences.

My freedom on the outside was nearly up. Soon I would have to face the drive back to 'Colditz Castle,' and its inhabitants. Bill was on hand again and, as usual, was full of encouraging words. Technically I was bankrupt. However, what I did have was an excellent support network via the hospital waiting for me on the outside. I also had a wealth of emotional support from four main families. After my second complete nervous break-down it had taken no less than 47 people to help put me back together again and 130 weeks in time. Seventeen months later I was to have a third bi-polar episode.

It was now 25 past six on a dark, damp Sunday evening as we approached the main entrance to 'Hitler Towers,' probably the worst light to see it in. All that was missing was the thunder and lightning and it would have looked like the Munster's house. The nursing staff you couldn't fault, although some of the young agency nurses couldn't give a monkeys about the patients. They had the power of the ward keys over us. It was their sole duty in life to make the mentally challenged amongst them wait 20 minutes for almost everything. Bastards. On the Tuesday following my so called 'successful' week-end at home I had my eighth and final ward round. I sat down in front of the usual crew, Trish, Dr. Gadhvi, a C.P.N. (community psychiatric nurse), a social worker and a trainee pencil biter and foot shuffler. I couldn't help notice there was a different air to the proceedings to that of my previous, "How are you feeling in yourself," ward rounds.

Trisha, it seemed to me at least, plunged in with her with her opening gambit and the only question of this short meeting. "How would you feel if we were to discharge you today?" In my medicated haze I thought she was talking to some else! I waited for the "Beadle's About" film crew to enter the room, but the door didn't open. Realising she was actually directing the question at me, my first thought was, 'she's having a laugh surely'. My second thought was 'shit, she is seriously expecting me to answer that in front of all of the people in the room'. I said in a child-like manner and a drugged stupor, "It's not a very nice place out there." Trisha turned to Dr. Gadhvi sitting to her right, and then looked towards me and said, "That is a realistic view from someone in your condition." I got the feeling that it didn't matter what I said, the exit from my bomb-proof sanctuary was a foregone conclusion. So I told them what they wanted to hear, though not exactly in the words they may have chosen. My delayed and sceptic reply was thus, "Well, I'll give it a go I suppose!"

Typically, I didn't feel ready for such a dramatic change to my routine. I imagine I was beginning to look too comfortable in the hospital environment. Trish continued, "We feel that it is important to maintain the momentum of your recovery." She was right of course, as she said, "The in-patient cycle had to be severed, sooner rather than later." But it sounded such a harsh comment after three and a half months of the kid glove treatment. I was asked if I had any definite plans once I was released. The sound of this question seeped into my thought process, and eventually my mouth formulated another child-like response. "I think I will spend two weeks at my Mum's flat in Berkhamsted to convalesce, it's nice and quite there. Then perhaps she could spend a couple of weeks with me at my place." "That sounds like a positive plan," Trish replied, "do you think your mother will be able to cope with the situation?" I thought, "I dunno, fancy asking me, I'm just saying the first thing that comes into my head!" But actually said, "I don't know to be honest with you, I'll have to ask her." "We know this must seem like a bit of a rush to you," Trish went on, "But we believe discharging you today will benefit you in the long-run."

Like a long burst of automatic gun-fire discharged in the Grand Canyon the word, benefit, echoed around my skull... Months back I recall Bill filling out my sickness forms for me. I hadn't in fact received a penny of my sickness entitlement during my 14 week stay in hospital. It was, as if I didn't feel bad enough, a terrible financial existence. I survived on donations sent by post from Mum, and Bill made sure I had a constant supply of nicotine when he came to visit me. I am indebted to both of them. My whole day revolved around where my next packet of cigarettes was coming from. That was my only requirement. At that point of this bi-polar episode I was smoking eighty a day.

Trisha interrupted the tail-end of the gun-fire, "So, we are all agreed, (nods of approval at the three desks in front of me), you will be discharged this afternoon. There will of course be a support network waiting to help you get settled in at home. I will give you the relevant paper-work when you leave later on today. If you want to you can phone your Mum from my office." I was in such a state of confusion when I ambled into the ward office that the nurse at the desk had to look up my mother's phone number for me. I think she was as stunned as I was when I told her I was being released that afternoon.

She told me not to worry and said, "Uncle Reg and I will come and collect you. Just give me a ring when you know what time you want picking up." It was now 11.30am, a Tuesday I believe. The process of being discharged, like everything else in Claybury, seemed to take forever to come to fruition. I spent the next two and a half hours trying to trace my elusive wedge from the hospital's benefit office. It was a nightmare. I was assured by the bespectacled Doris, (female clerk) behind the counter that, "This wouldn't take long; your money will be in the computer system somewhere." Dangerous words I felt. I took an immediate dislike to the words, long, system and somewhere. "Now, if you can just tell me your admission date, ward number, phone number, home address, your post code and your date of birth, I can begin?" She had to be fucking joking right! My brain collapsed and slipped down the back of my shirt and joined the rest of my bodily organs at the mentioned of my admission date. As I had more chance of squeezing a small blue whale up my arse than giving her this information, I went to look for one!

I returned to the ward office, beer vouchers in hand, all £670 worth. "That should put a smile on your face, Neil," a nurse said stupidly. "It's not going to cover three months mortgage arrears," I replied. At 2.30pm I said my goodbyes and thankyous as best I could and made my way down to reception. I heard the words, "Come on Bill, let's get you away from this place." I couldn't see the face as I was blinded by brilliant sunlight. But I new the sound and the warmth of that unmistakable voice. I should explain that Uncle Reg, who wasn't a blood relative, always referred to me, from birth, as Bill. I only questioned this point with him once in my twenties. My drinking partners couldn't understand why a family friend never called me by my christened name. Uncle said simply, "When Jeanne brought you home I leaned over your cot and said to your dad, that's not a Neil, that's a William if ever I saw one. I stood in a dishevelled repose. At my feet was a large grey plastic bag with Claybury Hospital emblazoned on it in bold black type. It might just as well have read,

"THE NUTTER HAS LEFT THE BUILDING"

The contents of which was the sum total of my three and a half month sabbatical from life as I remember it. There were my clothes, some clean, some dirty, some unworn, but all creased. A half eaten packets of mints, three wine gums, an assortment of sweet wrappers, Biros, virgin crossword books and the dust from the draw that they were housed in. On top and sticking out of my retards rucksack was a pile of hospital documentation I knew that I would never read. I was numb with shock and felt no where ready for this. I was leaving the hospital as I entered it, cold, fragile and scared to death. Why was I going home, I had nothing to go home to? Ahead of me all I could envisage was desolation and the likelihood of homelessness. I slowly poured myself into uncle's car, before I knew it I was standing in my front-room saying goodbye to him. Nobody informed me that I would be treading water for the next thirty months, and even then I would never fully recover from my second break-down.

CHAPTER SIX

<<<< THE LONG WAIT >>>>

Uncle Reg left saying, "Keep your chin up Bill, and take care." While mum made her way to the kitchen I stood in the middle of my front-room in a static, bewildered silence. I heard the pouring of water and the click of the kettle, and then a set of staggered flash-backs began in my head. What appeared in front of me was an abridged version of the events leading up to my second admission into Claybury. It was an awful home coming. People's faces zoomed in and away from my face. I could see their lips move but as before my tormented picture show had no sound track. The matinee ended abruptly when mum placed a mug of tea under my nose. I had hoped to feel better in my home surroundings. Instead I became too aware that I was floundering in my own environment. I was glad to be away from the 'fun factory,' but now I had the unenviable task of reasserting myself back into the community. Shaking off the stigma of Claybury was only ever going to be an up hill struggle.

I walked into each room of my lifeless abode, turned the water back on and checked the key meter for electric. Everywhere I looked I saw a future bill landing on the door-mat. To add weight to my financial dilemma, there, waiting for me, was a pristine white envelope. The letter cheerfully informed me how many thousands of pounds I owed in mortgage arrears to the nearest penny. I ran my door keys through my fingers and wondered just how long I would be able to keep hold of them. Technically I was already dead in the water. Thankfully we didn't stay long at my place. Mum had booked a cab to take us over to her flat. I couldn't wait to get there, I felt as if I was drowning in a raging negative sea. I can recall the pitiful and vacant feelings I held inside which I'm sure were visible on my grey, pasty face. I couldn't think for myself, I couldn't think full stop. My brain was a mass of confusion. I left hospital knowing I liked only two things, tea and cigarettes, three, if you counted sleep! That's was my base, that's what I had to fight my way back up from.

On Wednesday I woke up at the hospital waking hour but something was amiss. There was an absence of shouting, banging, white coats trying to rouse me out of bed and cold air and cold lino under foot. What replaced this cacophony of madness was a comfortable bed, a warm bedroom and carpet between my toes. This was most disconcerting. I blinked my eyes and waited to hear the familiar sound of a hypodermic syringe being placed in a kidney bowl, followed by the words, "Get some sleep now Neil." The view, feelings and peacefulness remained. As I hadn't blacked out I got up. Mum was still in the land of nod, so I bathed myself in the ambient solitude for as long as possible. The tranquil scene came to a close when the postman shot half a ton of paper-work through mum's metal letterbox. Mum got up and got dressed and the day began to unfold. This was the first time in 14 weeks that I had spent 45 minutes by myself. I was no use to anyone at this point. Not living as such just surviving because of the people around me. It's not a situation I ever felt or feel comfortable with. I was apart of other people's routine because I didn't have one of my own. I knew I had good cause for this but all the same, after a few months of mental and physical redundancy, I felt I was a burden to everyone.

The first 14 days spent in mum's ivory tower past all too quickly. I was hoping to feel a lot better than I did before returning to Chingford. In fact, unfortunately, I felt just the same as when I was discharged. Perhaps this was too much to hope for. My flat wasn't a safety zone. It was a holding bay for negative events, past, present and future. It reeked of unhappiness, but it was only me who could sense it.

The stark reality of my plight came to fruition when the next fortnight shot passed and mum returned to Berkhamsted. I have never known or felt loneliness like it before in my life. I sat in a pall of doom for hours not knowing what to do. All of the problems I had to face enveloped me at once. It is a pain I'll never forget. It's as if some had placed an anvil on my chest. I carried that weight with me for months at a time. I had all the time in the world but didn't know what to do with it. I now faced the daunting task of looking after myself for the first time in eighteen weeks.

Prior to my illness I had 24 years of routine, structure and financial stability behind me. All that had been obliterated now. I had lost everything to depression and four and a half months of psychiatric hospitalisation. I wish I had a pound for every time I thought, why me, what had I done? It was a waste of brain power. It was too late - it had happened. I was in my own personal Hiroshima fallout zone. I had no choice in this cruel twist of fate, and that is the hardest part to come to terms with.

After this second break-down, a bi-polar high, my thought process was badly damaged and I couldn't organise myself as I used to. My concentration was appalling. I couldn't focus on anything longer than a few seconds, so watching television was a complete waste of time. I was restless, irritable and bored stiff. But when someone suggested something to do I didn't want to do it. I didn't want to talk either; I knew all the answers to my questions. The days were long and tedious and I was racked with mental torment for weeks at a time. I presumed that this was what life would be like from then on, lonely, cold, confusing and introverted. I hated my new persona. It made me feel like a fourth class citizen. Adding insult to injury my acute melancholia had affected my spending power. Gone were the days of buying what I wanted; now I had to buy what I could afford. Except cigarettes of course, they still remain a priority today.

The day came when I finally had to go shopping for myself. To the uninitiated this might not seem such a big deal. But to a fresh, ex mental inpatient, the whole experience was as bad as being banged up for the first time. I needed milk, that's what got me out of the flat in the first place. I clearly remember looking in other peoples' baskets for inspiration because I couldn't remember what I liked to eat. When I realised I couldn't plan my meals for the next two days I had my first panic attack and had to leave the shop.

Having less money in my pocket than usual helped fuel my depression. Having said that a million pounds wouldn't have helped my recovery sad to say. The illness has to run its course. Gradually I got used to going into supermarkets again. Although the process did take me eight months. What's to get used to you might say? For me it was being in large building with people who were well. I felt so out of place because everybody around me had a grip on their lives. They could rush around making snap decisions on what to buy. Me, I was having trouble buying a packet of salt! There was too much to look at. Rows and rows of confusion was all I could see in front of me. The last daunting task to face was the check-out. If anyone was holding up the queue it always seemed to be me. The whole shopping experience made me sweat profusely from start to finish.

Through my depressed and heavily medicated eyes the aisles were marked up differently than they used to be. Instead of fresh meat, poultry or tinned fruit what I saw was totally different. The first aisle I encountered was marked, for the redundant man over thirty with a mental health problem, who had lost his job to technology and was now on benefits. In its abbreviated form these shops were named Pound Stretcher, Kwik Save or The Happy Shopper. This was to make the poorer customers feel they were getting the most out of their benefit money. In my experience these places should be called, No Choice Sucks, The Lard Emporium, or maybe TITOPYCATBFF. No, this isn't a foreign licensed bandit corner shop at the end of your street, it stands for, This Is The Only Place You Can Afford To Buy Food From! Again - no bloody choice.

Just passed the broken biscuit shelf I noticed a dark corridor marked, The Week-end Father Display Cabinet. Further on and deep into the bowels of the shop was a cheery aisle entitled, Single Parent Whose Friends Were Now Few And Far Between! I found no happiness in The Happy Shopper. No frills shopping meant no nutritional content, no taste and shit packaging. But hey, you only get what you pay for right!

I learned very quickly the reason hospital grounds are so palatial. I needed the massive expanse of space for its therapeutic value. It was the first thing I missed when I was discharged. I would wait until it had begun to rain then make my way to the forest that encircled Claybury. On prior walks I had found a few places where I could shelter. I sat by myself for as long as it rained; sometimes for two hours or more. I felt safe and snug in my little hideaway as I listened to the rain fall around me.

In the distance I could hear the speeding traffic of the rat race that I used to belong to. Not now though, the days ahead would be spent in solitude as far as I could see. It makes me laugh when I hear people talk about the space in their lives. Space to them means being in a different part of the house to the rest of the family. Well it's a start I suppose. Space to me means time span, isolation, and an ambient setting.

My first year on the outside was a trail in itself. I wasn't well enough to return to work and not ill enough to be in hospital. To a degree I wanted to be around people, but not necessarily to converse with. I had solitude in my flat but it was cold, unstimulating and full of bad memories. In the beginning I spent my days at Bill's house. That became part of my routine, get up and go to Bill's, I did that on and off for two and a half years.

Initially I wasn't allowed to drive because of the strong side-effects of my medication. After eight weeks the blurred vision, nausea, lethargy, diarrhoea and headaches had subsided somewhat. This meant I could drive to mums which turned out to be a pitfall that was difficult to get out of. Once I was there I found it hard to go back to the gloom of my flat. I would be at home for two days and want to return because I couldn't stand being in my flat on my own. It was a terrible sickening feeling that not everyone understands.

After three months of treading water I had the measure of my drugs, the side-effects of which were the same as a good session down the pub. The pub, my God, I had forgotten what it was like to sit in a bar with a pint of Guinness in front of me. I began a survey of pubs in my area that I had never drunk in before. Mainly because I wanted to drink, not talk. The embarrassment of meeting someone I knew was too much to bear at the time. Alcohol blotted out the pain I was in nicely, and helped pass the time. You see the loop-tape was still running only not as fast. Looking back I'm not sure which was worse.

However I had found a legal substance that stopped and ejected my cassette of problems, if only for a short time. Of course the next day it was up and running again. It's a hard cycle to break and can be dangerous if you drink heavily. Alcohol reduces the effectiveness of medication. I was in such mental and physical pain, a pain that is hard to describe, I continued to drink to numb my aching body. I drifted from pub to pub, in Chingford and Berkhamsted, thinking I was invisible in a crowd. It hadn't occurred to me that I stuck out like a dogs cock because I was a lone drinker. I regained my passion for playing fruit machines. Winning was incidental. Judging how the machine was playing was the biggest hook. It wasn't just an addiction. Mixed with alcohol, it was the perfect distraction from all of my worries. Don't get me wrong, I played to win. If I lost there was the next night's onslaught to look forward to.

I played the slots with a logical approach. The different combinations of winning entranced me for hours on end. More often than not I walked away with a pocket full of shrapnel (loose change), enough for a curry on the way home and plenty left over for the next night's session. It wasn't living, it was an existence. I did what I had to do to get me through another day.

In my drunken stupor I felt invisible and that way I didn't feel a burden to anyone but myself. I was putting the world at arms' length if you like but I felt I had to in order to survive. I had little to say, drunk even less so. How many solo drinkers have you met, that you didn't know from Adam, have you struck up a conversation with? See my point! People left me alone and at the time that's the way I liked it. Although sad, it was the only thing that I had any control over.

I felt a deep embarrassment for the people who new me, like I had let them down in some way. A chat with an old school friend would start, though I tried to avoid them, "High, how you doing?" "Not bad." I'd say lying through my teeth. "What you been up to then?" Like they didn't already know. "Oh not a lot really, been banged up in the local sanatorium for the last three and a half months!" I didn't know what else to say to people. The conversation stopped short about there. They felt embarrassed, I felt embarrassed, and the whole situation was so awkward. I didn't want to put people through that; I avoided them all for about fifteen months.

I had regular appointments with my surgeries C. P. N. (community psychiatric nurse) I am now an advocate of one to one therapy, it helped me in so many ways. I looked at it as talking medicine. It made a change to have something that didn't have a side-effect attached to it. On leaving Claybury I was still well below what was classed as the normal line and still had a few more rungs to climb.

Steve's first poignant sentences to me were, "There are no magic words I can say that will help you over night. But in time, and in conjunction with your medication, venting your feelings in this private room will be beneficial to you." He was right. He listened dutifully and was seemingly unshockable. He alone was responsible for the unravelling of my tortured mind. My opening gambit to him on hearing his first and an all too familiar question, which was of course, "How are you feeling in yourself at this point in time?" was, "I still wish I was dead, but I couldn't commit the act." We took it from there...

Steve's logical reply was, "That is your first rung up the ladder to normality since you were discharged." He had an uncanny knack of helping me understand a problem. Therapy is not a leaps and bounds process, you have to take that on board right from the start. But, if you only move forward an inch in that day; it's an inch further forward than yesterday. That's it in a nutshell. People who suffer from depression come to a grinding halt quite literally. Once you begin to pick up the pieces of your life again, and as long as you keep going forward, no matter how slowly, it's a positive sign of recovery. Hanging on to that basic theory and sometimes gritting my teeth got me through my second complete nervous break-down.

There is no doubt that depression tests the patience of the carers. Further into the illness you find out exactly who your true friends are. If you had a broken back or legs you would be either strapped to a bed or have a plaster cast, visible proof of your injury. After a designated amount of time the cast is removed and the broken bone has mended itself. I was walking and talking, sometimes, so what was the problem? Because I have a fluctuating illness people around me presume I now have a good day everyday, well I don't. Some days I don't want to leave the house or be with a large group of people. It is at this point of the illness where the uninitiated person's patience begins to wane.

People think because my break-downs occurred a while back spaced over 12 years that I should be fit enough for a full time job now, well I'm not. Three times I regained employment and every time I had another break-down. The stress on my wife and family is not worth a sixth break-down, so I have turned to writing. Because right now it is the one thing that I am good at. The most common thing said to me by people who don't understand me, normally children who I can forgive, is, "Why do you do everything so slowly?" Or, "You took your time doing that didn't you?" Oh please, tell me something I didn't know already. The thought of hearing these two comments said in a new work environment, with a room of complete strangers would crush me. I have to keep reminding myself it's me that's had five complete nervous break-downs. It's me that has had E.C.T. and it's me that will be on medication for the rest of my life. I have every right to be slow in thought. I may have regained most of my lost marbles but I will never be as I was.

Having said that, I am a more patient, diligent and thorough person now. I simply can't focus for long periods of time like I used to when I was at work. Because of my bi-polar disorder my concentration is sapped after an hour and a half per day. If you think it's frustrating to watch somebody who is slow, you want to try being me for six months! The overwhelming factor is what people don't have the patience for, or understand, they ignore, and it's the easiest option. God help them if a close family member suffers from depression. It's not so easy to blank when you see what depression can do to a person and a family. Some of my closest friends stopped phoning me after my second spell in Claybury. I have even witnessed people I know crossing the road to avoid me. I sometimes wonder who actually has the mental health problem!

Very little seemed to change in my life; the steps forward were so minute. I felt incompetent at everything. I knew friends and relatives were trying to help pump up my confidence but I only ever felt patronised. Steve called this the shooting myself in the foot period. He was right of course; I was beating myself up from the inside with the biggest stick I could find. This is a vicious circle to break. I couldn't believe I would be good at doing something ever again. I was wrong. It was no fun dragging my carcass through the day, but that's what I had to do in the end. Taking each day as it comes is fine for a while but I found it bloody frustrating not being able to plan anything in advance. Some days I couldn't get out of bed. Eventually I slipped into the, 'I'll do that tomorrow' routine.

Steve explained the importance of having a structure in your life, mine had totally collapsed. Above all else, if you have to start from scratch as I did, you need a direction, something to aim for no matter how small. As someone said to Bill once, "Aim for what is achievable and you won't be disappointed."

All I could see in front of me was the whole gloomy picture in glorious panoramic vision, and now there was a supplement to my loop-tape, the Pearl & Dean advert! It took at least 15 months to over-ride the daily thoughts of, what's the point, I will fail and it will all turn to dust in front of my eyes again. Everyday I climbed the greased pole and everyday I slipped back down to ground level. The main point was at least I was trying. In the end it was blind determination and sheer bloody mindlessness that saw me through each hour of the day. Steve gave no false promises about the future. The hardest comment I had to take on board was when he said to me, "Your medication will help up to a point, the other fifty percent has to come from you."

That was my worst meeting. I didn't know where I was supposed to draw the strength from. The more I looked for a quick answer to my abundant problems the less I found. I had to learn to let go of the things I had no control over, like the aggro with my mortgage for starters. Once you begin to accept that things aren't going to be as they used to, life becomes a little easier to cope with.

Without realising it I had stepped up another rung of the ladder but this part of the process really sucked. It meant I had to drop my standards. It was that or end up back in hospital again. At one of my countless evenings with Bill and Seron, Bill mentioned his mum needed a hand in her garden. He was to busy with his many outlets of work at the time. I had played in it as a child and it was easily big enough to get lost in. My first and typical response was, "I hate gardening." But then I hated everything at the time, even myself. A few days later I was making tea in Bill's kitchen when I noticed Joy struggling with her lawnmower. I leant over the fence and asked if she wanted any help. "Yes, she replied gratefully, "Would you finish mowing the rest of the lower lawn for me?" Mentally it was the best day's work I had ever done.

When I completed the lawn I stood back and looked at what I had achieved. Now it might not seem a lot to you, but, that freshly trimmed lawn looked like a work of art in my eyes. I felt so buzzed up I was cracking jokes and smiling from ear to ear. That was the first time I noticed a complete change in my mood since leaving the hospital. I was so chuffed with myself I phoned Mum immediately. She was pleased for me and so was Steve. After all the brain-dormant months it felt so good being of use to somebody. The emotion of achievement stayed with me for days. This was to be the start of my recovery and the beginning of a new structure.

Joy asked me to help out in her garden on a regular basis. It was only two hours a week but at least I now had a sense of purpose to my week. Up until that point everyday was the same to me. I had no division between the week and the week-end, except the Sundays in my life. You hardly have to open your eyes in the morning to know its Sunday in England. Although gardening wasn't my ideal pastime it turned out to be both a therapeutic and an educational time. Joy had hundreds of plants and knew all of their names. I had all the space I needed and could relax in a tranquil setting. It was a pleasant feeling to be able to lose myself for a while from the outside world. I could also take note of the wild-life that rented Joy's garden. I can vividly recall in the depths of my depression not being able to appreciate a hot summer's day.

Ted, Bill's dad had recently died, and more often than not I would sit and talk to Joy long after finishing up in the garden. For a short time at least I found an inner peace there. Bill's sister, Anne began making enquires about my services. In no time at all I had something to do every Monday, Wednesday and Friday. Anne's house stood in three quarters of an acre of land so there was plenty to keep me occupied. The bonus for me in the height of that summer was a swim in their outside pool and why not, I deserved it. After the battering my brain had taken this form of convalescence was exactly what I needed.

From then on I decided to concentrate on feeling better about myself for a change, rather than worry about small pieces of paper with the Queen's head stamped all over them. Money won't stop a break-down occurring or help a millionaire recover. It was now one year after being discharged and all I could cope with was six hours of light duties a week. But at least I was doing it. My confidence began to improve alongside this new structure which, in turn, enhanced the value of my self-worth. Then, as now, things still take me a long time to complete. Something as simple as writing a cheque out for a bill can take me twenty minutes. I can't concentrate if people are watching me either, I feel too self conscious. It is the legacy I am stuck with after my break-downs, but it could be worse.

My meetings with Steve became farther apart, I saw him once a month instead of once a week. I no longer thought of death as an answer to my problems and my new medication had reached its therapeutic level. It took 15 months to get the right mix of tablets that suited me. Not many people understand how time consuming getting the right anti-psychotic medication can be. Bill had kept tabs on my progress and one day asked me if I fancied helping a friend of his out. Cautiously I asked, "How do you mean help exactly?"

Alongside Bill's estate agent work he ran a building contractors with a mate of his called, Graham. He explained that Graham was a man down on a local job and wondered if I would like to lend a hand. Seron chipped in, "He's a really nice bloke, you'll get on well with him." Both Bill and Seron were good at planting a seed and watching the idea grow on me. With my usual non-committal approach it took a week or so before I agreed to meet Graham and we hit it off straight away. I was nervous of meeting him because he was the first new person I had met since leaving the 'fun palace.' Bill had clued Graham up on my illness and said that it wasn't a problem. All the same, even after 12 months I still felt uneasy around strangers.

My psychiatric past didn't faze Graham at all. As it turned out his brother had a long history of mental illness so he new roughly what to expect. He was openly saddened by his younger brother's depression and, like many people, didn't understand the illness. Graham and Roger had worked side by side for years and he had witnessed first hand how depression had ravaged Roger's life. "Compared to 'im," he said, "You're a walkin' miracle. Rog' stumbles about like a tit in a trance most of the time. The Doc' says the drink is 'alf the problem." I sympathised with Graham and recall vividly being in the same awful zombiefied state myself.

Tentatively I asked Graham what I would be doing. He replied, "A bit of this, a bit of that and a bit of fetching and carrying. What do yer reckon then, up for it or what?" What was I supposed to say? For a start, there were too many grey areas for me, I needed clear, concise guidelines, but there comes a point where you just have to jump in with both feet. I mentioned to Graham that my biggest fear was working with a whole new bunch of people I didn't know. In fact the thought terrified me. "Well," he said scratching his beard, "it'll probably do ya some good." I was afraid of making a prat of myself. Graham assured me that my medical history was known only to him and Bill. "Fink about it for awhile, if yer interested give Bill a call." "That's the problem," I said, "If I think about it for too long I'll talk myself out of it. There was a pregnant pause and I said, Oh bollocks, when do I start?" "Tuesday," he replied.

Before he left Graham asked to see my hands. "Bit soft, office worker was yer?" "Oh please," I said sarcastically, "Printer, man and boy." "You mean had a licence to print money and never done an 'ard days graft in yer life", he said winking. "Yeah something like that, shame the gravy train's in the sidings now." "As long as you've got a pulse, I've got some graft you can 'elp me wiv. We'll soon 'ave a few decent blisters on them for ya." I could see the day looming when the kid gloves would be pulled off and thrown on the incinerator.

I was soon to learn that what Graham didn't know about the building trade could be soldered to a piece of fuse wire. He had the obligatory workman's bottom, which was evenly balanced out by his rotund beer gut. His wise cracking frame was a welcome change in my life. What started out as just lending a hand for a few days turned into working five days a week. It was a real boost to my confidence; I was doing it, actually doing it. I even regained my sense of humour, which seemed to be appreciated. Just making someone laugh made me feel so much better about myself.

The two trades couldn't have been more different. The laughs on site centred around quick bum, tits and knob jokes. A joke or wind up in my trade could take up to three days to come to fruition. Education was at the route of this division. That may sound a snobbish accusation to throw around, but having said that, you still need brains and an education to build a house. The main difference between the two trades was the physical effort required. The building trade is not for the faint hearted. In short, it's the most backbreaking way of earning a living I know. I was a thirty three year old apprentice, and yes I did feel like a prize prat to begin with. My calluses and blisters blossomed nicely when I rose to the dizzy heights of mixing up sand and cement. One of my hardest day at work consisted of feeding three bricklayers with mortar and cement for three hours solid. I have never worked so hard in my life. A month had passed by and Graham checked over my hands again. "That's a bit better," he said. "I'll make a builder out of ya yet. 'Ow do yer feel?" "I'm absolutely fucked thanks to you!" "That's the game," he said, and with that he walked away whistling to himself. I didn't like labouring I just got on with it, and working in the elements, mostly rain, wasn't much fun. I was too used to a nice warm building rather than the great outdoors. I was either wet, cold or covered in crap or a combination of all three. But the summer months more than made up for the drudgery of winter, when I was hot, sweaty and covered in crap!

I spoke to Graham on a number of occasions about how depression had affected his brother and himself. I could see the frustration in his eyes. "It's a crying shame, he said, "He used to be so on the ball, such a laugh. Now he just walks about in a world of his own." Some of you will have heard this comment before, Graham said he felt like shaking Roger in the hope that he would snap back to how he was. If only it were that simple. Like the symptoms to the patient, the sayings of the carers run parallel with the illness.

The bad news kept hitting my doormat and I began to slip into a low spot again. I was also worrying myself to death at the prospect of getting back into my trade. I had been out it for so long by then that the new technology was fast leaving me behind. I wanted what I couldn't have, my old job back at D. S. Colour. I went to the same place for twelve years, it was my second home. In effect I was grieving the loss of my long-term employment. It was just one of the crutches that were kicked from under me, it didn't exist anymore.

My appointments with my CPN were increased to once a fortnight - I was stuck again. Steve decided to change my medication as he thought it wasn't working with me. Today's anti-psychotic medication still seems to be a hit and miss affair to me, but that is all we sufferers have available to us. For the patient concerned, their life is on hold whilst the correct drug and dosage is prescribed for their particular branch of mental illness. For me this only led to more frustration. As with depression the side-effects are also invisible. Everyday for weeks at a time, I faced a dry mouth, nausea, lethargy and blurred vision. Initially the stronger down-side to my medication included: diarrhoea, vomiting, muscular spasms, trembling hands, restlessness, a broken sleep pattern rounded off with hot and cold sweats. Notably all of the above affected my social confidence.

To reach its therapeutic level, you have to be taking the medication for at least two to four weeks. Waiting for something to happen made feel me so irritable. Bill and Graham understood my predicament and I took some time off from the site work. I stayed in touch with them both and returned to my gardening duties. It seemed par for the course that every time I hit a low spot I received a truck load of paperwork from the benefits office. More explaining! They always arrived on a Saturday, so you couldn't phone them even if you wanted to. Phone them, that's a laugh. The last few times I have tried to contact the benefits office the annoying recorded voice told me the opening and closing times, followed by all the bank holidays in Europe! Then I was informed that my call was held in a queue with a waiting time of twenty-eight minutes. I slammed the phone in disgust. I got the same reply three days in a row.

I'm sure they were in league with my mortgage lender, because their letters arrived at the same time. I know they were only doing their job, these faceless people, but I felt as if I was solely responsible for paying back the national debt. I didn't open them straight away; they either contained bad news or seventy-two pages of stuff I couldn't make any sense of. On the whole I think that the benefit agencies, such as the CSA, make the genuine claimant feel worse, suicidal in some cases. I made my extra trips to the doctor's for the relevant paperwork regarding my health on countless occasions. This only compounded my depression. Not only was I redundant, I was ill as well. It is a terrible combination to fight your way back from, but not the worst. I new someone who was an alcoholic and a manic depressive.

As if my life wasn't bad enough, my benefit office wanted to know when I would be fit to return to work. At that point I didn't realise I had a fluctuating illness. I used to feel incensed when I received their letters. I wanted to scream at them, "Leave me alone, you're making me feel ten times worse than I already do." To this day I am quite sure that the people who work at these offices have no idea how a computer generated letter can crush a person.

I heard of a case through a friend of mine who worked on Equilibrium with me. It seems an ex- inpatient received 15 letters in one day regarding arrears on his council tax. Like most of us, he couldn't bring himself to open the doom-ridden post. He was in such a state of panic he barricaded himself in his house for six months. Eventually he was evicted. You can't claim benefits unless you have an address. He was on the streets and living rough for months before finally being re-admitted to hospital. Subsequently he got back into the benefit system and was re-housed. But what about the countless others who aren't so fortunate?

From time to time I was summoned to my benefits office to check if I was actively seeking work. For the most part, as I said, I was concentrating on my well-being, not that anybody I ever spoke to understood that or my illness. Instead of what was supposed to be a personalised service, I only ever felt victimised. I didn't seem to fit in their cubbyhole of clientele, the dead and the living!

I was walking and talking, so I must be fit for work. Ah, that old chestnut. They didn't have the time quite frankly, the minute you mention the D word they ask you to send them the relevant paperwork from the doctors I mentioned earlier. So I filled out the forms that they wanted me to. You know, the ones that remind you of what you've got. How many break-downs you've had? What wonderful hospitals you've had the pleasure of staying in? And, how long you've been redundant? All that sort of cheery stuff! I felt as if I was lying to them, like I had brought this illness on myself. As if I hadn't had enough of my character stripped away by redundancy and ill health, there was another kick in the bollocks to come. When I informed the college leaver who was interviewing me of my earning potential he quipped, "Aah, you may have to think about lowering your sights on the wages front." What he actually meant was, a shit job equals shit wages. I wasn't about to be pushed into a dead-end job, just so that he could massage the unemployment figures to the tune of one. At this point I begged the question, "How would I pay my mortgage and arrears on £175 a week?" I used to earn double that. The meetings used to peter out at this point.

There were plenty of courses to go on if you had the confidence to learn something new, but I didn't. In the late eighties finding new employment was hard going. There were carpenters re-training as electricians, electricians attempting to be printers, (thanks to Maxwell, Murdoch and Thatcher), and 'plumbers and brickies' swapping jobs too. As tradesmen none of us would be headhunted. We, the cannon fodder of the work force, just had to get on with it. It took me an immense amount of time to accept that the printing trade, as I knew it, had disintegrated. I thought I had a job for life. Thanks to depression I was stuck in a time-warp and couldn't visualise myself doing anything else.

The benefit office's next stratagem was to encourage me, and I use the word encourage in the loosest terms possible, to visit a job club. The word I would have chosen would have been blackmail in every sense of the word. The letter I received stated that my benefits might be cancelled if I did not attend. So I popped along to the shabby looking building in Walthamstow. This was far more depressing than group therapy. There I met a bunch of unemployeds who looked as pissed off as I felt. The guy in charge swore blind he could cross-reference our existing jobs into new ones. I didn't believe him for one moment; neither did anybody else there that day. What I needed to do in hindsight was to integrate back into a working environment, and not simply jump straight back into full time work.

My illness set me apart from the majority and should have been treated as such. After all, how many employers would have taken on a person with a mental health track record, let alone integrate back into work? I felt I couldn't mention my illness to people I didn't know. I've seen the unnerving looks on their faces too many times before. You would think I had something contagious. Look one says, is he going to go off and attack someone and glance two says, is he safe to be around children! I'm afraid to say that the mental health stigma is alive and thriving in the year 2006. My CPN put me in touch with an organisation called Quest, which was funded by Waltham Forest Council. Although it took me three months to summon up the courage to phone them I was glad when I did, they were so helpful. It was a user run group which was such a relief because they new exactly how I felt. They had been set up to help people in my situation. At last I felt as though I had someone batting on my side. They specialised in helping mental health users reintegrate back into work, helped with benefits problems and set up job placements and college courses. They would approach firms and explain the situation; in essence they were educating employers about the perils of stress and mental illness in the work place.

CHAPTER SEVEN

<<<< BACK TO THE RAT RACE >>>>

I did eventually summon up the courage to phone about a couple of jobs that I had seen advertised in the 'Daily Mail.' Bill helped me to revise my CV, and on paper at least I looked a pretty good catch. Like most trade jobs there were no in-betweens in your personal skill. You were either good or bad; bullshit didn't cover you for very long in the print game. If you were sloppy in your work methods you would have been sussed out in the first 15 minutes. Fortunately after completing a five year apprenticeship, two years later I could say I was competent at my job. But this was all before my first two break-downs had shattered my confidence.

Throwing caution to the wind I sent off my CVs and forgot all about them. Secretly I was hoping that no one would reply to my applications. I had been out of work now for two and a half years. Deep in my heart I knew I couldn't cope with the going back to work process, it was going to be too much too soon. I just felt that I owed it to the people around me, like my Mum who had supported me through thick and thin, to at least try.

What Bill, Seron and Mum didn't know was that the thought of a new job, new people and a different routine all at once had made me physically sick. I received a phone call one day from a firm that I had sent my CV to. My heart sank. The bloke I spoke to sounded really keen and wanted to set up a meeting as soon as possible. I tried to make all sorts of excuses for my time off work in a desperate bid to put him off the idea, but he talked me into a corner. I now faced an interview in central London. In a blind state of panic I phoned Bill to see what he thought I should do. The details of the vacancy sounded attractive, if you were of sound body and mind. I wasn't at the time and I had a bit of paper to prove it! I arrived at Bill's house ten minutes later and found him sitting in his back-room, calculator in hand. "Come on then," he said, "hit me with the details?"

The wedge is 20 grand a year, four nights a week, 6.00 p.m. to 6.00 a.m., plus five weeks paid holiday, plus double time over time." Bill punched in the figurework and, as positive as ever, said, "Financial problem solved. With the overtime on the Friday that's a possible earning capacity of twenty-eight big ones." "Yippee," I replied, trying to sound enthralled with this news or though clearly I wasn't. After speaking to the guy on the management side, I was told that the night manager would also like to speak to me. I gave Bill's phone number as I wanted some support around me when he called. He was going to phone that night, Tuesday, at 10 o'clock, so I had all day to churn over the prospects of the job. The more I thought of a return to work, the more the idea repulsed me. I was hoping that the bloke I had spoken to first might have copied Bill's phone number down wrong, no such luck. Bang on 10.00 p.m. Bill's phone rang.

"Oh… bollocks," I muttered to myself, trying desperately to push my heart back down my throat. I made my introductions and half way through his second sentence I said, "Can I stop you there for a minute, is that Geoff, Geoff Frazor, ex of D.S. Colour?" "Yes," he answered, who's that there then?" Stumbling over my reply I said, "It's Neil, Neil Walton, we worked together in the plate room at the mad house." He remembered the name but couldn't put a face to it. This put a completely different slant on the whole going back to work malarkey.

It must have been about eight years since we last spoke. I asked Geoff what the firm was like to work for. "Usual story," he said, "the blokes on the bench are okay, it's management that haven't got a clue. The money's good but they do want their pound of flesh." "So it's nothing like D.S. then?" I asked hopefully. "Unfortunately no." I felt my heart making another bid for freedom via my windpipe. There was a long pause when Geoff asked what I had been up to over the years. "Mostly being made redundant," I finally replied. "It gets more popular every year," he quipped. My overall fears were that I hadn't worked for ages. Also this was a night job, four twelve-hour shifts in a row. That was a forty-eight hour a week to start with, on days at D.S. I was only doing a thirty-five hour week. I should have read the signs and said no to the job, but like a fool I said I'd see him on the Monday after the interview with his man in the office. It was shit or bust time. As I put the phone down Bill said, "Well, good news or bad news?" "A bit of both really." I replied. "I know the night manager from D.S. Colour and the money's good but it's a pressure factory."

I was shaking and sweating, and that was just talking about the job over the phone. I should have called a halt to the proceedings there and then. Instead I did the exact opposite to what my mind was telling me to do. In true depressive style I back-catalogued my way through a stack of problems to come. Could I do my job came top of the list? I knew then it was the wrong move to make. Bill shouted from the kitchen, "So what are you worried about then?" "How long have you got?" I replied.

Monday came around all too quickly. I hadn't used public transport for so long that I had lost all track of the cost of the fares. I arrived at the desolate over-head station in plenty time. Only to find that a machine had replaced the human being that used to give me my ticket. I had no change; this was just the start of the daytime nightmare. Like the White Rabbit in Alice in Wonderland, I dashed to he nearest paper shop, changed a ten pound note and ran back to the station. A train had just pulled out.

Getting a piece of card with my destination stamped on it wasn't going to be as straight forward as the instruction label said. I aimed a hand full of pound coins in the metal monster that was disrupting my travel plans. After frantically stabbing away at the buttons nothing came out, not even my money. Another train pulled in. I read the instruction again and again; I was looking but not seeing. It might as well have been written in Gujarati for all the good it was doing me. The train that had recently arrived, departed. I got the feeling that the machine was enjoying this game. It stood there with a quiet happy buzz flashing its small red light at me. I'm sure I heard it laugh! Now I had two would-be commuters standing behind me. Bucket loads of water began to pour from every sweat gland in my body.

"Having trouble," one bloke asked? "If it was a fruit machine I would have sussed it out by now," I said mopping my brow" "Where are you going," he inquired? "Oxford Circus." "Return." "Yes," "Sling £4.80 in and push those two buttons." The ticket machine whirred into action. Four seconds later out shot what I had been trying to get hold of for the last 40 minutes. Shortly after that out came the change I thought the machine had eaten. A third train entered the station. The relief of getting a ticket was unbelievable. I couldn't thank the bloke enough. My nerves were in shreds long before reaching my destination.

I changed at Walthamstow and made my way down to the Victoria line. The minute I entered the bowels of the tube station I had a vivid Claybury flash back. The echoed noise of the trains and the bustle of the travellers in the tunnels were identical to those of the corridors in the hospital. Panicked, confused and disoriented I made my way back up to the over-head section of the station. As I lit my first cigarette a train pulled in going back to Chingford. I watched as it left and disappeared into the tunnel and wondered why the hell I didn't get on it. I ummed and aarred as to whether I should continue with the rest of the journey. I had had enough already and wanted to return to the safety of my life-less flat. It was only going to get more crowded and noisier the nearer I got to Oxford Circus.

I kept telling myself I had to beat this fear and eventually stepped on the tube heading towards central London. I couldn't believe that people put themselves through this form of travel everyday. I had done it in the past and didn't bat an eyelid, but I didn't have any mental health problems back then. It wasn't a train it was a cattle truck. It was a horrendous ordeal for me to go through. Someone who has suffered a complete break-down, has had just that and it affects everything that they used to do. The nerve shattering experience, in my view, is on a parallel with First World War shell shock.

Despite the gap in using public transport, one thing remained the same. I noticed you still had to pay even if you stood up for the entire length of your journey! My trip was no exception. I claimed my place on the carriage in the upright position near a door. Praying that when it was my stop, and my turn to prise myself away from the heaving mass, the platform would be on my side of the train. In the past I have seen grown men and women locked in hand to hand combat trying to get on and off this wonderful form of transport. As the train picked up more and more people I was hemmed into a corner. For the next seven stops bad breath, cheap perfume and straphangers' armpits surrounded me.

The tube pulled into Oxford Circus. As the doors opened I was faced with a platform full of commuters. Now you would think the most logical approach in this situation would be for the people standing on the platform to stand aside, allowing the passengers on the already full train access to disembark. Even the bloke on the Tannoy System agreed with me. But no, the game was to push and shove until a fight broke out. It seemed that courtesy went out of the window and the train doors when it came to getting home in the evening rush hour. Having been pushed from pillar to post and back again I fought my way towards the escalator. A tube pulled in at the opposite platform and a seething mass joined my trainload of would-be escapees. It was sheer madness. I was surrounded by power walking, brief case carrying, brolly toting morons. I wondered then as I wonder now, who was actually the sanest person there that day? I knew - sadly it would be years before they did. Suddenly Claybury didn't seem so bad after all.

The more I looked for an escape route, the less I saw an appropriate exit. I hitched a ride on a moving staircase. This seemed to be all part of the game, it was moving and most importantly, it was moving upwards! Thinking I had left the power walkers far behind, to my left, they had been replaced by power stampers. These prats were actually running up an already upward bound escalator. This was the most ludicrous thing I had seen for along time. When I reached the top of London Transport's free ride for the war-torn traveller, I could see why they were in such a rush. The next hurdle, and I use the word in its fullest capacity, was the queue at the ticket barriers.

I witnessed grown adults throwing themselves over this obstacle like lemmings, rather than wait in a semi-organised fashion. The first thought that entered my head as the static menace sucked the ticket out of my hand was, would I ever see it again? It had to give it back it was a return. No it didn't! My sweat glands primed themselves for another workout. I felt the huffing and puffing of an impatient crowd of power walkers breathing down my neck. Obviously it was my fault that the ticket checker eaten my pass. I looked feverishly for a railway employee and eventually a guard braved the baying mass and retrieved my travel card from the machine. I found an exit that lead me up to street level. I left one thronging mass of people behind me, only to join another out side the station. There was no escape.

Everywhere I looked there were crowds of people, eating, drinking, walking and begging. I found a doorway that wasn't occupied, which is rare in Oxford Street, lit a cigarette and gathered my thoughts. I leant back and took in the view of this human version of a disturbed ants' nest, knowing shortly I would have to join it. I got the feeling that at least a bunch of ants would have been more organised.

I had a short meeting with the manager of the firm. I told him that I had been redundant for sometime and briefed him on my past work history. "So you know Geoff then?" He inquired. "Yeah, we worked together at D.S. Colour." As many people did, he seemed impressed with the name, D.S. Colour, and the fact that I had worked there for over 11 years. "Geoff should be in soon, he informed me, is there anything you want to know?" I dare not ask him how much work I would be expected to produce. I replied, "No I don't think so, my only fear is that I've been out of the game for so long I think I may be suffering from ring rust." "Don't worry," he said, "I'm sure we'll get you back on track." This sounded fine in practice but then the words, 'pressure factory,' rang in my ears.

At that point Geoff stuck his head round the office door. "Long time no see," he said with a cheeky grin. "How's it going?" He then proceeded to show me around the various departments. Things had changed so much that I didn't recognise my own trade anymore. Straight away I noticed the total lack of atmosphere about the place. It was a head down, key pressing, mouse clicking, sterile environment. And, there was a general absence of apprentices to set a light! What used to take six hours to produce manually, now only took thirty minutes with the aid of computer technology. This meant that the person at the end of the chain producing the quick proof for the customer, i.e. me, would be swamped with work. I must have been mad, my entire body and a large part of my brain said, don't take the job but I did. As I said, I felt I owed it to those around me to at least try this job out for size. In a moment of calm I remembered something a journeyman said to me before I joined D.S. Colour. "If it all goes wrong," he said, "just remember, they can't shoot you." Seventeen months later I would have quite happily shot myself! I should have listened to my gut instinct, but everything hinged on the wages of this job. I will never put myself in that position again. My health and sanity are far more important.

I checked out the equipment in my department, most of it had been up-dated. I spent a twelve-hour shift at a friend's firm. They had the same of machinery that I would be using, it gave me a rough idea of how it worked, but I only picked up the basics in that time. I hadn't given much thought about what it would be like to work on a night shift. It took four agonising months for my body clock to get used to the change round from day work to night work. In those initial months I didn't know when to eat or sleep. This was dangerous territory for anybody over a prolonged period of time.

The first week had to be the worst four days of my entire life to date. By the end of my shift at 6.00 a.m. on the Friday, I was having trouble keeping my eyes open and standing up. I was asked in I could go in for 12 hours over time on the Friday. I declined their kind offer of the extra cash, which didn't go down to well with the management. I dragged myself to the tube station. When I reached Wathamstow's windy over-head platform I arrived just in time to kiss a train goodbye that was heading for home. I could have happily curled up and died there and then. Twenty minutes later I boarded a Chingford bound train. I was dog-tired, staving hungry and freezing cold. My legs and hips hurt so much that it took me twenty-five minutes to walk to my car which was parked out side Bill's house. Normally the walk to the station took me about ten minutes. As I lumbered my way towards my vehicle I noticed it was covered in a thick layer of frost. I couldn't be bothered to scrape the windscreen; I didn't have the strength or the inclination. So I sat there for god knows how long until the heater had done its work.

At 7.40 a.m. I arrived home. Nothing was going to stop me crawling into my bed now. I thawed out in front of the grill cooking my breakfast. I struggled to pull my clothes off but by 8.30 a.m. I was under my duvet, safe in the knowledge that I didn't have to go back to work until Monday evening. I didn't drift off to sleep; I passed out and woke up twenty-three hours later. I came to at about 7.30 on Saturday morning wondering what happened to the last day of the working week. Sleep deprivation is something that I hadn't thought about properly. At best I was getting about five hours sleep a day.

The muscles in my body had been out of a work routine for some considerable time, I ached in places I didn't know I had places. Sunday disappeared in a blur of tiredness, and before I new it I was back at Chingford Station, fighting with the ticket machine again. The minute I walked in the firm on Monday evening I was jumped on by one of the office staff to see if I could work on the coming Friday. I found myself saying yes to things that I should have been able to say no to again. I got known as, nervous Neil, not only did I feel like shit, people were laughing at me behind my back. I kept telling myself that I had to keep going no matter what they thought of me; after all I needed the money. The firm itself was modern and clean and the guys on my shift were a nice bunch of people. But overall it was run by the exertion of fear and pressure on its workers. The only thing the management staff was concerned with was a quick turnover and a high profit margin, and they didn't care how they got it. Can't perform; get a new bloke in, that came from the top. By the mid nineties man power was expendable and my trade union didn't have the clout that it used to have.

By the Wednesday of my second week I was beginning to flag, and the thought of doing the extra hours on Friday played on my mind. I was dead on my feet but I went in all the same. The biggest shock I think was the workload. In the past, at D. S.   there were natural breaks during the day when things went wrong and work had to be returned to various departments. I now faced a forty-eight hour week over four nights, 60 hours if I worked on a Friday. I blinked and missed all of Sunday, and the start of my third week was upon me before I knew it. I was asked if I could go in on the following Friday and again I said yes. After a month of this work cycle I was under a black cloud and back to the doctors to up the dosage of my anti-depressants.

I couldn't tell anybody at the firm about my appointment with my CPN, or ask for time off, as I hadn't been there long. On that day I only managed to get three hours sleep and I had to skip breakfast. Prior to all of the above I received a call from the manager who interviewed me. He wanted to know if I could start a week earlier than was agreed. Originally I thought I had two weeks' grace before I had to face the awful first night nerves. I said I had a few loose ends to tie up with the benefits office before I could start but he didn't buy it. In fact he began to get stroppy with me saying that he had got people covering my shift and I needed to start as soon as possible. He talked me into a corner again. It seemed he was all right as long as he got his own way. I know, I know, I should have told him to poke the job where the sun don't shine, even my CPN showed some concern. Steve remarked if the job becomes to much for you give it up, at least you have tried your best. But then I would have had to face all the hassle with the benefits office again, which I'm sure you will agree is a forbidding experience in its self. No, I was determined to make a go of this.

Have you ever had one of those days where everything you touch falls apart in your hands? Well that was exactly what my first night was like, pure hell. The evening started off okay, the journey in was less fraught for starters. I even purchased my ticket from a human being. Sadly that was the best part of the whole night. I hovered outside the firms' doors for a few minutes before entering. As I walked down stairs everybody I passed turned round and looked at me as if to say, there goes another lamb to the slaughter. I was in a state of confusion before I got to my small department. What I actually wanted to do was put my coat on and make a quick exit; there was no escape now. I was stuck there until 6.00 a.m. the next morning; I would have rather gone over the top at Flanders.

As soon as I took my coat off, I was jumped on by a member of the production team. He wanted a two-colour proof knocked out as soon as possible. When I took a closer look at the job specifications, the colours that the customer required were both special colours. This meant they had to be applied by hand not with the aid of machinery. It wasn't a problem except I didn't know where the special colours were kept. When the guy asked me when it would be ready, stupidly I said, twenty minutes. Twenty minutes later I still hadn't located the special colours. When I did find them, there where pots of hand mixed colours everywhere. They should have been marked up with a reference number. At least this would have given me half a clue as to what the colour was supposed to be. Only about a third of the pots were marked up properly. Geoff explained to the now frantic office bod that I had only just started working there and didn't know the run of the place yet. He picked out two colours and said, "Slap them down, they'll do for now." Twenty minutes later the job was complete and I breathed a sigh of relief. I couldn't remember when I felt more stupid.

I returned to my department to find six job bags on my bench, all marked urgent. Another bloke walked in and said, "Drop what you're doing and slip this one in before you start anything else, there's a bike courier booked for half an hour." I went looking for Geoff. When I explained the situation he went and had a few quite words with the bloke concerned. I heard the tail end of the heated exchange of words from four yards away. "Don't jump all over his back, it's only his first fucking night." Geoff returned to me with a pleasant smile on his face and remarked, "Don't worry about all that, they all try that on, you'll get used to it." The last thing I want to do was to start making enemies on my first night. I pulled the four colour film separations out of the bags in front of me in a bid to look like I knew what I was doing. Realising I didn't, I made my way to the little boys' room. I had lost the power of concentration due to a severe panic attack.

When I returned to my department I was greeted by another member of staff, with a smile and four more job bags. With a deep sense of embarrassment I went looking for Geoff again. I explained I was dying on my feet and some more work had turned up and I didn't know where to start. "Okay," he said, "I'll be down in a minute, don't look so worried." As I walked past the production bench I overheard one half of a phone conversation. The bloke my end said, "Four colour proof, right. Special gold and silver, yeah, bike courier, three quarters of an hour. Airport, DHL Germany yeah, yeah no problem." "Oh… my… God," I thought, "surely they aren't going to give that to me?" I was about to commit hara-kiri with my scalpel when I heard the news that the advert concerned

142

had been cancelled. By the end of my shift I had a nervous twitch from hearing the words, special colours.

A few minutes later Geoff stuck his head round my door and said, "How you doin' then?" I replied, "Well I've been here two hours and so far I've only managed to knock out one piece of work." "That's life," he said with a daft grin on his face. "What do you wanna know?" I pointed to the mess of films and job bags on my bench and frowned. "Aah, you need a running order don't you?" "Right, put that, that and that, up with that. "One four colour cromalin, cyan, magenta, yellow and black. Piece of cake." At last I had something in front of me that I understood. All I had to do now was get it through the new machinery. My nervous twitch kicked in when I thought about the ticket-buying escapade before I reached my interview. Geoff was called to the phone but before he left he said to me jokingly, "You know your trouble..., you worry too much!"

I laminated a piece of cromalin board with its light sensitive coating and positioned up the cyan positives. After exposing it in a vacuum frame to artificial ultra violet light, I pulled off the blue films and tore back the top layer of laminate. With everything crossed and filled with hope I offered the board up to the ATM (automatic transfer machine), and pressed the go button. There was a God after all! The board shot through the machine and came out the other side. I pulled back the waste cyan colour sheet and was left with my first colour intact. After a short prayer I repeated the sequence in readiness for the second colour. I pushed the go button, stripped off the magenta top sheet and some of the cyan image and most of the magenta came with it.

I binned it before anybody noticed and started again. The same thing happened. Before I had a chance to dig a hole and jump into it, two more job bags turned up, both with special colours. I sidled past the production bench and hid in the toilet. If anybody else said, how's it going, I think I would have burst into tears. I had no option but to find Geoff and relay my tale of woe, making sure the management staff were as far away as possible. Geoff, as placid as ever, came and watched me start the job again after I showed him what had happened to my first two attempts. He remarked that there might be something wrong with the colour rolls on the ATM.. I said, "What, you mean this has happened before?" "Yeah, sometimes the stock is knackered before it arrives. It might be an idea to make a note of the batch number; I'll check it out later. Just remember, not everything that goes wrong is your fault."

The blue and red went through without a hitch. "There you go, it's a breeze." He said. I prepared the board and patched up the yellow positives. I don't think Geoff had been gone more than two minutes when I discovered the yellow had stripped off the first two colours. I was lost for words. At that point I was about to tell Geoff about my break-downs but the more I thought about it the more it sounded like a poor excuse. Countless other opportunities occurred through the night where things went wrong but by 4.30 a.m. I was too tired to care. I apologised about my poor performance profusely, "It's your first night remember," he reiterated, "stop apologising, tomorrow's another day." "That's what I'm worried about." I said, "See you tomorrow." Geoff replied, "Don't you mean tonight?" My heart sank when I realised he was right. I was a night worker now which meant I had to get home, eat, sleep during the day, get up and go straight back and do it all over again. I suffered acute anxiety attacks for over twelve months before my drugs were changed yet again. Finally after seventeen months of working a night shift I had my third break-down.

CHAPTER EIGHT

<<<< OUT OF MY MANOR >>>>

I was spending the weekend with a former girlfriend and her daughter. It wasn't until the Saturday that I realised I had forgotten to pack my medication. At the time I was on a maintenance course of anti-depressants, just a hundred and fifty milligrams a day. I didn't think there was much to worry about. How wrong can you be? I missed seven tablets in all and by the Sunday midday I was on a massive high again.

I was playing a tape of my old band's music, quite happy in a world of my own. The tape finished so I put on a record called Eric Clapton Unplugged. The record played through and I was fine until a track called 'Tears in Heaven' came on. I just sat there listening to the lyrics and began to sob. This went on for entire length of the song. I remember screaming when it faded out, "You bastards, I want my Dad back the way he was," tears still streaming down my face.

Some of this episode is sketchy so you will have to bear with me. Apparently I went to the kitchen, picked up a carving knife and started waving it about. My girlfriend and her daughter fled the flat. The scary thing was I don't remember a thing about brandishing a knife. Gill phoned Bill and it was he who contacted the police and forewarned them about my illness. I was still listening to some music in the front room when there was a knock on the door. I went to see who it was, and standing there were two police officers. They must have asked me who I was but can't recall hearing any of their conversation. Although, as high as I was, I do remember speaking to them but I haven't a clue as to what I said.

I was now face down on the floor outside the flat being searched for the knife but I must have left it in the flat somewhere, because the two officers didn't find it on me. The light frisking only lasted few minutes then I was allowed to stand up. When I did I noticed groups of policemen standing in two's and three's, with two more standing on the metal staircase above me outside Gill's flat. Altogether there were seventeen officers present.

Feeling a little more than crowded, I slipped into my Tai Chi routine to keep them at bay. I tried to escape up the metal staircase but I was pulled down by the back of my jeans. I went over to the wall that surrounded the tarmac area, and looked over to see how much of a drop there was. It was about 40 feet to the ground - too high to jump. I turned round and faced all of the officers while the two coppers that had knocked on the door earlier tried to talk me down. I remember trying to get back in the flat, saying I needed to go to the toilet, but two coppers just stood there blocking the doorway.

The next thing I knew I was in handcuffs and in the back of a police wagon yet again. I have no recollection of the journey to the hospital and I don't recall getting out of the wagon or being un-cuffed either. I was now in a long corridor saying hello to anyone that walked past me. Another time lapse must have occurred. I was now in a dimly lit room with just a mattress for company. I was sitting on the mattress when in came four men in white coats, followed by half a dozen policemen. I had no idea where I was or what I had done to be in this situation. I was hoping by now that I would have forgotten all about these nightmares but I still see them. These events occurred ten years ago. I wonder if this would be classed as post-traumatic stress now.

What made it worse was one of the chaps in the white coats produced a hypodermic needle and said, "We need to give this injection to calm you down. Will you allow us to do that?" I shrank back on the mattress with my back against a wall with ten unknown faces and a needle staring at me waiting for a reply. I must have said yes because I remember undoing my jeans. "Before you give me the jab," I said, "would you promise me that you'll phone my friend, Bill." "Yes, of course," one of them assured me. The policemen stood back and I laid face down on the mattress. I pulled my jeans down to my knees and the nice young men in their clean white coats knelt down and held my arms and legs in position. The injection was administered without a struggle. After the jab everybody left.

My next reference point was that it appeared to be daylight again. Christ knows what was in that injection, presumably something to drop my adrenaline rate I guess. Well, it did that all right - it also blotted out six days of my life. I was sectioned for twenty-eight days under the Mental Health Act, but only stayed in Hillingdon for seven days. Things may have worked out differently had I been transferred back to Claybury, which is where my medical records were, and where I was first admitted with clinical depression. I guess that the council budget didn't run to that expense.

Five months later I was still suffering the side-effects of the injection. My partner at the time said it was like going out with a different person every time we met. Sadly the relationship ended. She is a recovering alcoholic on a twelve-step program with Alcoholics Anonymous. She also had a daughter to bring up, and there was me with a few problems of my own. It was just a bad mix. Subsequently when my mother informed my firm that I had been sectioned for twenty-eight days, I was sacked because all of a sudden my work wasn't up to scratch. What a strange coincidence?

On my next jaunt in Ruislip, for some reason I had got it into my head that I was on a physical training course, now completing the last section which was road running. The fantasy started to kick in. I was in the Para's. I began to pick up the pace but still not knowing where I was headed, I began looking for signs of which direction to take next. I saw a car indicate left so I went left, then a lorry indicated and turned right and so did I. This went on for a mile or so. After that my signals for direction became less organised. A Coke can in the road go left, a stick on the pavement, go right, you name it, I followed it. It was then I noticed a road sign for Northolt Aerodrome - the fantasy in my head was now complete, but took another path the second I saw that sign. I was now in the RAF.

The airfield was at the top of a gentle incline but still about three-quarters of a mile away. By now I had pulled my shirt off and was running as fast as I could towards the air-base. I was chanting to myself, "Got to get to the top," repeating it over and over mantra style. Finally I made it after running roughly three miles. I then collapsed in a heap outside the gates of the airfield. A guard came out to see what was wrong. I was too exhausted to speak. It took me ten minutes before I could stand up and get my breath back. At this point I noticed three more guards coming towards me.

I shouted, "Just leave me alone, don't touch me, I want to see a face I recognise." To add to my predicament six military police joined us. I still couldn't work out what all the fuss was about. At this point I should mention, Northolt Airfield is used for the Queen's plane to land. Unfortunately I was in no fit state to recognise the problem I was now causing. The guards and military police must have thought I was a serious threat to her Majesty and the country as a whole. I said to the bloke with the gun, "You're going to need more than that the way I'm feeling pal." The young guard didn't move a muscle.

After my second breakdown I took up Tai Chi, Yang style. This was for relaxation purposes. Relaxing it was, but, used for self-defence, it is lethal. My armed escort couldn't have known that I had only just completed learning the form, which involves fifteen minutes of continuous movement and takes nine months to learn, so I played on it. I was now surrounded and shouting, "Don't touch me or I'll take you all out." I knelt down, picked up two rocks and held them to my head. I recall thinking I'd kill myself before they got hold of me.

I was backed against the wall of a long building. They were gradually edging me along this wall towards a rubbish area where I could be cornered. I was now standing in front of a single brick-width perforated wall, which looked like a large waffle. I moved two more paces to the left and stepped backwards to find I was trapped. There where some dustbins, old bricks, rubbish, and a pair of step ladders in one corner. I put the ladders up against the wall and could see that there was no escape. I began to punch the wall with the palms of my hands and had removed about a dozen bricks in this way forming a v-shape. The guards and the military police moved in closer. They where trying to distracted me by calling and shouting to me. I don't remember what they said exactly but it worked. As I turned round to speak to the guard on my left, one of the other guards grabbed the back of my jeans and pulled me off the wall. I dropped eight feet to the ground into a mass of sticks, leaves and loose earth.

I was pinned face down and handcuffed. For some reason, now I was trussed up like a turkey and no threat to them, they started to hit me repeatedly. Beginning with my calves, upper legs, then lower and upper back, shoulders and arms, they seemed to enjoy this part of the chase as I heard one of them say, or rather shout, "Go on, do it some more, he's mad, he won't feel it." I would dearly love to meet them all now and have a quiet word, just to put all of them straight on a few points. On reflection I have often wondered how many times ten people can hit a person in five minutes? Quite a lot I should imagine, especially if you have a stationary, bound target. I remember screaming at the top of my voice, "Enough, enough, you bastards." The beating stopped. I was dragged to my feet and led away. I looked like a fox that had been pulled through the undergrowth for an hour by the hounds. Sometime later a police wagon was sent to pick me up.

There isn't much room in the back of a police van. The rear section allowed seating for two with a thick Perspex interior panel, separating driver and passenger from their cargo. This compartment is used for difficult or violent people. There is a gap in the middle section of the Perspex panel top and bottom. This allows air to circulate throughout the vehicle. I knew what was coming next but I was powerless to stop it. After a while it begins to get warm in this compartment. It was a hot day anyway, and this only sped up the effect on me. You start to feel drowsy and weak because you are deprived of fresh oxygen, after twenty minutes you're nice and pliable.

When we arrived at the station a side-door was opened for about five minutes. There was a nice rush of fresh air to my brain and it was as if I were drunk. When the back doors were opened I got another blast of fresh air that topped up this drunken feeling. Still handcuffed the police officer helped me out of the van, sat me down on a stool and after a few minutes gave me some water. We stayed outside in the open for ten minutes or so before entering the police station. I was booked in, seen by a doctor and then put in a cell. It was semi-cool and serene at last. After the pandemonium beforehand I was now in total isolation. The silence was deafening. So quiet in fact, I could actually hear the blood pumping around my ears.

Even in my dazed, clockless world, it was clear to me that I would be there for quite some time.

I stood with my bare back against the cold steel door, it was sheer bliss. To pass some time I walked in circles punching three of the four walls. I couldn't reach the fourth wall as the bed in the cell prevented me. This went on for quite sometime, half an hour or more. I then sat down in the middle of the cell floor, blood seeping from my knuckles. I stared at the only source of natural light. A window made up of glass blocks six inches square and I guess three inches thick. There were forty-eight to be precise. I remember counting them over and over again out of sheer boredom. I couldn't see much through these blocks as there was an irregular moulded shape in each one. After a few moments I got up from the floor, knelt on the bed and with saliva on my forefinger I daubed a huge crucifix on the cement between the blocks. I watched as the cross slowly began to evaporate in the heat of the now humid cell.

My concentration was broken by the sound of people in the other cells calling out to the duty officer for things like drinks and cigarettes. I was gagging for something to drink myself but I couldn't pluck up the courage to shout for anything. At the age of thirty-eight this was the first time that I had been arrested, let alone placed in a police cell. Why was I here if I hadn't done anything wrong? I realise of course that I was, probably, a danger to others and myself. But, was the Queen landing at RAF Northolt on that particular day? Answer, I think not.

When I remembered I couldn't remember the last time I had had a smoke, I lost some of my inhibitions and thought, fuck this for a game of soldiers, I need a fag right now and started tapping on the door with my fingers. I built up a nice rhythm too, but I didn't get much attention from anyone so I began to hit the door a bit harder. I have been a drummer for many years so I could keep this up for ages. I think the plan was to make as much noise as possible, for as long as possible, so the duty officer would have to let me out. In hindsight they must have heard it all before. I kept the percussive solo up for a long long time, hitting the door with my feet, knees, fingers and fists. This opened all the wounds on my knuckles from punching the cell walls earlier. I eventually got the attention of a duty officer and got a cup of tea.

Before he brought it into my cell he asked me to sit on the bed, which was opposite the cell door. This put a safe distance between us, giving him enough time to put the tea on the floor and re-lock the cell door. He asked if I was okay and if there was anything else I wanted. "I'm fine I think thanks," I replied, "but I could murder a fag right now." "I'll see what I can do," he said. I asked him how long I had been banged up. "Six hours," he answered. Just before he left my cell the police officer said, "You won't be here much longer, a friend of yours is coming to pick you up." The door was locked and he went back to his duties. I racked my brains trying to work out who was coming to collect me. I couldn't remember any of my friends or family names, except one, Mum…

Sometime later there was a rap on my door. The policeman had returned with a packet of cigarettes and another cup of tea. "Bless your little heart," I said in thanks. The officer smiled a wry smile. "Same procedure as before," he said. I sat on the bed and waited. I was dying for a cigarette. The constable put the tea and cigarettes on the floor and locked the door behind him. Then I thought to myself, hang on a minute, how am I going to light the bloody things, I haven't got any matches? All of a sudden there was a loud clunk. A metal plate a bit bigger than a letterbox was removed from the cell door. It was then that I heard the sweetest sound of the day, the click of a lighter. I heard a voice say, "Could you put your hands behind your back please?" Shit, I'd have chopped them off if it meant getting hold of a fag any quicker! Putting the cigarette in my mouth I walked over to the vent. The policeman, still taking no chances, lit the cigarette at arm's length from the outside of my door and then disappeared up the corridor back to his work.

I wasn't allowed to keep the lighter for obvious reasons. So there I was, with twenty cigarettes only one of which was alight. I protected it like a baby. Inhaling three large draws of smoke I rolled the tailor made cigarette around my fingers, gently blowing the amber tip to make sure that it didn't go out. They weren't my usual brand but I didn't give a toss, nicotine never tasted so good. It wasn't until I had smoked over half of the cigarette that I remembered I didn't have any means of ignition in the cell, (A heavy smoker's nightmare). I quickly lit up another from the pack and stood it on end on the cell floor so it wouldn't burn so fast. (A heavy smoker's survival tip) I used this as a taper, and then smoked two more cigarettes' one after another to top up my nicotine level. This procedure was repeated a few times while I made my second cup of tea last as long as possible. At a rough estimation I had gone without my usual fix of fags for over eight hours. My bipolar high had lasted more than eleven hours. At about half past eleven or twelve at night my cell door was opened. I was almost free. What a glorious feeling that was.

A policeman ushered me out of the cell and into the corridor. It had really bright yellow walls with blinding white florescent lights on the ceiling. It had taken me a few minutes to get used to it after the grim lighting in my cell. I was checked over by the doctor who had seen me earlier before being released. If the truth was known I was still a little high, but not enough to be detained any longer. Looking back I was still a time bomb waiting to go off. Finally I saw a face I recognised; it was my old schoolmate, Bill. He was without doubt my guardian angel and mortal sprit guide throughout the blackest period of my fluctuating disorder, not forgetting his wife, Seron of course. I had a lump the size of a Granny Smith in my throat. I beamed at him and he said to me, "Hi mate." To which I replied, "No, not at the moment although I have been for most of the day!" He just smiled back at me, gave me a hug and informed me there was a pot of tea and some hot food on the go back at his ranch. I don't remember any of the thirty-mile journey home, or who cleaned me up after the incident at the airfield. I just counted myself lucky that I had such good friends around me at the time and also how sympathetic the police were towards my illness.

After a few days had passed I ask Bill who dropped the cigarettes into the station. It turned out that on that particular day/night none of the officers on duty smoked. A WPC made a special trip to a garage and bought me some with her own money. It would be good to meet her one of theses day to say thanks in person. This particular episode you have just read took me over eight months to piece back together. Some of it came back to me in the form of flash backs which still haunt me today. The rest of it was like doing a five thousand-piece jigsaw, with conjunctivitis and no picture to follow.

CHAPTER NINE

<<<< PARANOIA >>>>

Do you remember 'proper' T.V. programmes like the Avengers or the Prisoner? Where things appeared normal to everyone except those people in the leading roles. This is fine in a half-hour episode but has it happen to you in a real life situation?

My first scene opens with a drink in my local. The minute I walked into the pub the atmosphere felt somehow disjointed. The interior decoration hadn't change, there were no new fruit machines and the phone, and cigarette machine were in their usual places. So what was wrong? I mulled it over with my first beer. A mobile phone rang in the next bar with one of those pathetic rings. I heard a voice say, "Yes he's in and just bought his first drink," finishing the brief call by saying, "yeah no problem I will, bye." Nothing too odd about that, until I realised that I was the only person my side of the bar. What made it worse was I couldn't see this person face. After a few silent moments I dismissed it as a coincidence, he must have been talking about somebody else.

A few minutes later I could hear two people talking behind me. I couldn't hear everything they were saying but as their conversation tailed off I heard one of them say, "Neil's in tonight, we'll have to keep an eye on him." I froze. I wanted to turn round to see these peoples' faces but thought better of it. I tried to convince myself they were talking about another Neil, which washed for a while. The bar had started to fill up now; it was then I noticed the next oddity of the evening. Not one of the people in my side of the bar were regulars. Come to think of it, it was unusual for me to be drinking by myself, especially on a Friday night. I breathed a heavy sigh of relief as I heard the voice of one of my drinking partner's, Jack, entering the bar. He had brought a friend with him that I hadn't met before. I wasn't in the right frame of mind for making small-talk with a complete stranger. I let Jack do the introductions and hoped that they would keep the conversation running, while I stood back pretending to listen.

When Mark went to the toilet I asked Jack what he did for a living. "He's a copper," he replied. "He's just been made up to a sergeant." "Oh right," I said, trying to sound pleased for his friend. This bit of information confirmed something else that had been bothering me. All of the people there that night looked like ex-servicemen or off-duty policemen. I scanned the bar once more because I was still hearing my name mentioned periodically, which by now was making me feel really uneasy. Still in listening and looking mode, I spotted the next quirk of the evening. There were no women in the pub, not one, not even behind the bar. The more I looked the more things I found wrong with the whole scenario. I was just about to make a quick exit when three of Marks work-mates turned up to help him celebrate his promotion. Another round was ordered and a drink placed in front of me. My escape was thwarted; I felt I was now being held in the pub by a tremendous social pressure magnate, which at that point I could have done without. The conversation in our crowd turned to the subject of the masons and my ears pricked up.

We had the usual jokes about the funny handshakes and the rolled up trouser legs of course, followed by an in-depth talk about this secret society. I managed to ignore the fact that every time a mobile rang I heard my name and focused all of my attention on what Mark and his friends had to say. Being in the 'job,' many of their senior officers would have almost certainly been attached to a lodge. It seemed the case that you were asked to join the masons, rather than approaching them for application. All of them had their own beliefs and stories to tell but none of them I thought were in a Masonic lodge, as they all seemed too young for one thing. I had my own thoughts on the subject. With considerable effort I managed to shut out the background noise of the bar, to reflect upon my own experiences. And I was still able to nod and smile in the appreciate places within in my groups' conversation.

Although my dad wasn't a mason, he belonged to a royal golf club. Nothing too strange about that you might think, except there is a Masonic lodge near every royal club in the country. When I left school dad thought it would be a good plan for me to get an apprenticeship in one trade or another. He asked a friend of his at the club for his advice. He in turn knew a friend in his lodge that worked in a printing firm. I'm sure you can see where this is going; low and behold I got my apprenticeship. Which was a real surprise to my careers teacher, as she told me that I wouldn't get in the print trade unless a member of my family was already working in a printing firm. In 1974 it was still a closed shop business - halcyon days.

Looking back, I felt covered in many ways, even outside of my parental guidance. As if I was being nudged towards a particular path. Especially between the ages of seven to twenty-one when I finished my apprenticeship in 1978. Had the things I achieved up to that point in my life, which I put down luck, coincidence or fate, been mapped out for me? When I thought back, most incidences could be backtracked to a friend of a friend who knew my dad or someone at the Royal Epping. This revelation shattered the elusion of my own self worth. Job offers that came my way, girls I had gone out with, even down to the school friends I knew. Had I in fact actually achieved anything off my own back or had I been helped along every step of the way? My concentration was broken by Jack nudging me saying, "Neil, Neil, the lights are on but is anybody at home, it's your round bub." "Sorry mate, I was fathoms away." After handing out the drinks, I made my way to the toilets to think things over in peace and quite. I locked myself in one of the cubicles and racked my brains for some answers to the night's strange events. Somebody came in after me and then I heard a mobile ring again. "Oh Christ," I said under my breath, "no, no don't say my name." A deep voice echoed around the tiles in the men's room and said, "Yes he's still here, yes, I'll see you soon." At least I didn't hear my name mentioned, but I was still convinced that the call was connected with me. I waited until the toilet was empty before re-joining Jack and the extras for act two. There was still something amiss with the bar scene, as looked around I spotted it.

Nobody was smoking except me, and I was the only person with an ashtray. Even Jack was without his usual cigars. To in-force this fact, I noticed there were no ashtrays on any of the tables and none on the bar, except the one that I was using. This was getting too weird for words and I now felt that everybody was looking at me. The last straw was realising that as Jack, Mark and his friends spoke to each other, I was listening to three separate conversations, on various subjects, all at differing speeds and making perfect sense of everything that was said.

I began to feel faint. I heard another phone ring just behind me, my head was burning and I felt a huge rush of adrenaline course through me. To make things worse as I looked at people's faces, they began to zoom in towards me, as if their necks were made out of rubber. I was now in a cold sweat and my head felt like it was on fire. I left my beer on the bar and headed for the pub garden to try and cool down. I remember feeling like this before. I was going high again. Had I halved or missed my medication? Probably, didn't know, couldn't remember. From past experience I knew anything could happen now. The frightening parts about my highs are that I don't remember the things I do or say until about six months later… Or unless somebody jogs my memory. Most people in the street would think I was a crack addict or just another drunk out to cause trouble. Failing that you are immediately put under the category of 'nutter, loony or psycho.' But in all cases – never ill!

After some deep breathing exercises I managed to pull my self back together. Returning back to the bar I necked the rest of my pint and ordered another one straightaway. The alcohol slowed down my adrenaline surge but what was I going to do when the effects wore off? To try and give you an example of just how powerful my highs are, it's like taking fifty amphetamines, (speed), one after another. To add to my problems, although I didn't know it at the time, I was having an acute paranoid attack as well. It was as if I had eaten a side plate of magic mushrooms.

All my muscles started to tense up, my libido becomes incredibly high during these periods and all my senses are heightened, aching, begging to be employed. I become overly confident, sharp and I feel dangerous. I leant up against the bar lapping up the sensation of internal power that had come to haunt me again. Unfortunately with this Jeckel and Hyde transformation I become verbose and lairy with it. I wasn't quite up to the walking on water stage yet. Although I have been there when I was prescribed Prozac by my doctor, but that's another chapter by itself. I had the good sense to walk out of the pub before getting into or starting any trouble, as I'm only in charge of ten percent my actions when high.

Certain sounds and words seemed to fuel my paranoia in the pub. Policemen, for one, with the exception of Jack and myself I believed that everybody else must have been in the 'force.' And just the thought of anything relating to tobacco stopped me dead in my tracks; I don't think I smoked more than three cigarettes the entire evening. The last word helped me formulate a conclusive answer to the night's strange events, the masons. Now the speed and magic mushrooms had been fully digested I convinced myself that I was being initiated into the masons. But to pass I had to be seen, publicly and privately, to have given up smoking.

High and paranoid the, 'what ifs' enter your head. What if they've bugged my flat? What if they've installed hidden cameras or microphones while I was out? The more I thought of a 'what if,' the more I thought things were going on behind my back. As I walked home the only place I could think of that might be safe was my garage. I opened the up and over door as quietly as I could and went in. As I shut it behind me I was plunged into darkness. I didn't care I felt safe and also much calmer. I sat on the floor fumbling for my cigarettes and lighter. At the end of my fourth cigarette my sanctum of peace was invaded by the droning of helicopter blades cutting through the inky blackness of a damp October night. I could hear people running through the car park shouting. By now the helicopter was right above me scanning the car park with a powerful searchlight. As it flashed through a gap in the garage door I moved to the back thinking if it touched me they would know where I was hiding.

I cowered in the corner and hid under my coat to muffle the noise, as gusts of downdraft battered the metal garage door. It was like being in a wind tunnel. The noise reached its peak, and then slowly subsided. The helicopter seemed to go straight up and disappear out of earshot. The car park fell silent. I moved towards the gap in the door, lit another cigarette and waited patiently to make sure the coast was clear. All appeared to be quite, just a hint of a breeze rustling through the trees that surrounded the flats. Gingerly, I opened the garage door and saw my car in its usual parking space. All was still peaceful. As I walked towards it I couldn't believe what I saw. It appeared to have four new tyres, hubcaps and two new bumpers. I took another glance around before getting in, and sat there in disbelief. My head was full of why's, how's, and what ifs. I assumed that I must have passed the initiation test and this was a form of reward from the masons. I lit a cigarette to celebrate, then realised I was now in the open so I ducked down under the dash board in case anybody saw me. After a couple of minutes I thought, sod this for a game of soldiers and sat bolt upright, still holding my cigarette down by the hand-brake. I opened the window to let some smoke out flicking my cigarette butt out at the same time. As I did this the dashboard started to move and contort. The clock started to change position and reduce in size and extra dials appeared out of thin air. I sat there motionless, as a new interior manifested itself in front of me. It was on a par with some of scenes the from Steven King's film, Christine.

I touched it once it had stopped moving to see if it was real and it was, well to me anyway. I thought that this was a bonus from the men in the black suits because now, I was smoking. I lit another cigarette just to see what would happen, holding it up in clear view through the windscreen. As slowly as it started the dash began to revert back to its original shape. "Oh cute, very cute," I said out loud. "They want to play mind games; well they had just picked on the wrong bloke." I had picked up a Ph.D. in, not being had over by anybody when I did my apprenticeship in the printing trade. Leaving the car, I checked to see if the other spare parts were still there but they had vanished as well.

As I entered my flat I did a military style search, bursting through doors and rolling over on the floor. As I got to the bathroom all was quite. I had checked out each room for people now it was time to look for any bugs that might have been installed. In the wall behind the toilet at head height was a small hole that I hadn't noticed before going out. "Very smart," I muttered under my breath. The bastards have planted a camera but why is it in the toilet and why aren't there any microphones? It took me a while to figure it out but I did eventually. Then I began to wonder which flat they might be watching me from.

I had families living either side of me, above and below me. I convinced myself it was a surveillance team working for the masons keeping tabs on the victim of their mental warfare. I came to the conclusion in my paranoiac state that they must be in the flat below. There were no microphones in my flat because the floor creaked when you walked on it, so they could tell if someone was in. Not only that you could also hear the toilet flush up stairs and their bath water running away. Obviously the same applied for the people in the flat below me.

I slide down in a corner of my front room and made sure I kept away from the huge window. Opposite my flat was a parade of shops with accommodation above them. I couldn't take the chance of being seen from that vantage point, these people might be armed. I sat there chain smoking, starring blankly into space for God knows how long trying to work out what to do next. I looked down at the floor at one point to find I was surrounded by cigarette ash and butts that were all burnt down to their filters. I checked my badly crushed packet to see I was down to my last two cigarettes.   Searching my pockets, I found a screwed up fiver and some loose change.   Ten minutes later at 2.00 a.m. the supply had depleted. Now all I had to do was brave the outside world to get some more. I lived near a busy cross-road. The only vehicles around at that time of the day were the odd police car or lorries heading for the M.25. It was the latter of these that concerned me the most. I crouched in the hallway gasping for some nicotine.   The nearest supply was just a hundred yards away.

I started to crawl along the hall on my hands and knees trying not to make the pine-flooring creek under my weight. I broke out in a hot sweat as another flood of adrenaline coursed through my body. Half way up the hall, I started to see flashbacks of the Iranian embassy siege, where the S.A.S. used sensors on walls to pinpoint people in a particular room. I wondered if this was really happening to me. The perspiration was running down my face, off my chin forming a small puddle near my left hand.

In a moment of rationality I stood up and said out loud, "Get a grip you prat, nobody shoots you for smoking." I Then casually walked out of my front door, sauntered down the stairs and made my way through the flats and out to the main road. The fresh air felt good on my sweat soaked face. I leant on the set of railings that led up to the traffic lights on the cross-roads to the left of me. I watched them change a few times soaking up the tranquil scene before making a move.

I had a choice of garages, one either side of the lights. As I walked towards them I noticed they had static cameras on top of them. Presumably these were for traffic control, but in my mind that night they were for keeping a check on my movements. So I strolled down the centre of the road with the intent of goading who ever it was into some sort of challenge. Not a murmur. "Tossers," I shouted at the top of my voice as I walked through a red light and stood bang in the middle of all four traffic lights. I turned right at a forty-five degree angle and ambled into the overly illuminated fore court of the petrol station.

I could see the attendant was on the phone and thought there and then that the call was about me. As I neared the counter we made eye contact. I cut him in half with a psychotic stare that a laser scientist would have been proud of. Within a couple of seconds he couldn't look me in the face, at that point I heard a vehicle pull into the garage. This was too much of a coincidence for me, it was a police car. I broke my gaze from the bloke's forehead, changed my body language and started to act subserviently. "Could I have twenty Lambert and Butler lights please," By now the policeman was standing right behind me. I could hear his radio crackle and hiss with messages.

I could see his reflection in a window opposite the counter that ran behind the cigarette cabinet. He was trying to get the attention of the garage attendant by putting his hands together at his chest height, then opening them to his body's width. Even I knew what this meant. It was a form of communicating to some one on a live T.V. broadcast. The signing meant; 'stretch out the commentary.' The copper repeated this a few times and pointed to his mouth before the bloke understood what he supposed to do. I resisted the temptation to say, "He wants you to engage me in a bit of banter, so he can work out what my mental state is like you plank." But I was to busy enjoying the reflected Ad break and watching this poor bloke squirm.

He started by trying to make small talk with me and said in broken English and I quote. "How zit goin' mate, vut is der vedder doin' out dare gore blimey, it's a bit blowy isn't oh yes." Well, I had to bite my lip hard to prevent myself from bursting out into a fit of laughter as these words came tumbling out of his face. I just raised my eyebrows a couple of times, smiled politely and teased my fingers over the sweet rack. I saw the policeman sign to the Indian guy again. The poor bloke broke out in a sweat not really understanding why the policeman was intent on keeping me there. This was starting to wind me up and I'm sure the policeman could sense it. It seemed I would have to play the game a little longer if I was going to get my hands on some nicotine.

 My body was craving the drug so badly now, that if I didn't get my hands on some soon I would have quite happily trashed the garage shop and the people in it. This is exactly what the policeman was waiting for. I wasn't going to give him the satisfaction, as I was mentally much stronger than he thought. The only thing the Indian guy could do to prolong my stay was to say he hadn't got enough change in the till. However, I was well ahead of this situation.

"Oh lummy!" He exclaimed, (wait for it, wait for it) "Vaunt you know I haven't got enough change in the till from a fiver, oh blimey, no I don't." "That's all right," I said grinning like an adolescent who had just lost his virginity to his French teacher, "I'll see if I've got the right money!" His face dropped as I looked pointlessly for money I knew I didn't have.

I was now internally seething but still managed to withdraw into my resource of staying ice cool. But much more of this sodding about and I would have exploded into the Jack Nicolson character from the film, The Shinning. The policeman knew how much pressure he was putting me under, but he just stood there in silence. Having said, that he wouldn't have had enough training at Hendon to have worked out a psycho like me, I had to many years on him. The atmosphere was so heavily charged in the shop you would have needed a chain saw to cut through it, rather than a knife. I had three ploys left open to me. I could have said, "Don't worry mate, I'll try the next garage," which of course would have put this poor bloke out of his misery. By now, he must have wondered why the constable was so intent on keeping me there for this amount of time.

Was I a mass murderer on the run? Or had I escaped from the local funny farm? Not this time around. These questions and more were written all over his face, at one point I actually thought he was going to faint. Ploy two was simple. Give him the fiver and tell him to keep the change but that would have sounded too desperate, too suspicious and too easy. I glared at him square in the eyes again, changed my body language and I put both hands on the counter. I was right on the edge now and in danger of turning into the cartoon version of the Tazmanian devil.

But this would have given the copper just the excuse he needed to nick me. I waited, almost bursting to use my final stratagem, within a millisecond of thinking of it I had changed character and said politely, "Couldn't you use some of the change in those money bags over there?" Earlier I had noticed a huge pile of coin bags stacked up against cigarette cabinet. There was a pregnant pause as the Indian guy looked at the policeman in the hope of some verbal support. None was forthcoming. I had outwitted the copper, making it one nil to me. The Indian attendant sank to his elbows on the counter, with his head bowed down.

The situation had reduced him to a nervous wreck and I was still feeding like a vulture from his mental weakness. He said, "Oh surely, I vas forgetting about dat monies, oh yes I vas, oh deary deary me." I winked at him in thanks for the cigarettes and change. He breathed a sigh of relief as I put them in my coat pocket. As I turned to make my exit, the policeman moved up to the counter. We never made eye contact.

His mate was still sitting in the patrol car with the engine switch off, clocking my every move. I stepped of outside the garage shop and walked slowly out onto the fore- court. I strolled past the car towards my flat inhaling huge lungfulls of cigarette smoke as I went. When I was a safe distance away I stood in the centre of the road again and in a fit of defiance I suppose, threw all my loose change high in the air. As the money clattered to the ground around me I did a Michael Jackson dance twist and went up on my toes. As much as to say, 'take it out of that you bastards.' When I heard the police car start up however I decided it would be a good time to make myself scarce, in case they followed me back to my address.

Maybe I had pushed my luck too far. When the rush had subsided, I felt the need to debase myself. I felt I had been too cocky earlier in the garage. Now I had to find a punishment to fit the crime. I ran a bath, a cold one. I had no heating in my bathroom so to make it even colder I opened the window. I kept telling myself I had been to smart for my own good so I had to knock myself down a peg or two, before somebody else did. As I stepped into the metal bath, remarkably, the water felt hot on my skin this was too good to be true. I even checked to see if I had used the correct tap. As I lay back in what was seemingly hot water I thought that perhaps 'they' didn't want me to humble myself to that extent. I reached for my cigarettes and as I inhaled the first draw of smoke a shock ran through my whole body. In the time it would take a snake to strike its prey the water turned ice cold. The shock to my heart was incredibly painful and I dropped the cigarette in the bath.

This was a heavy-duty mind game they were playing. The only way I could have felt something that was supposed to be cold but was in fact hot to the touch, was if I had been hypnotised. Now there's a thought from the 'what ifs' collection. But how was it done? It must have been a buzzword or sound in the pub. My straw clutching, as you can see, was getting much worse although to me all my thoughts were rational and plausible. Moments later of course I came up with a solution.

Every time I heard a phone ring in the pub I started to feel strange. Obviously it was the ringing tone that put me in some form of a trance. This wasn't over by a long chalk. Sod what 'they' wanted, I still wasn't happy with my performance in the garage and still felt as though I had to make myself suffer a little while longer. I decided to stay in the freezing cold surroundings and watched my breath drift up towards a light that was on the outside my bathroom window. It still amazes me how quickly my body adapted to the cold conditions. I had created a mind block against the temperature, putting every ounce of brain energy towards the subject of the Buddhist faith of all things.

I didn't know much about their faith I must admit but these people all ways seemed to be so peaceful and in tune with life as a whole. Maybe I was hoping to draw something from their beliefs. Any tasks I had to perform now would be done in a slow, methodical pace. I believed I was conserving my internal power to the point where I fully believed I wouldn't need to sleep, just rest, which I managed to do for seventy-two hours. As I reclined in the freezing water I was mind, body and soul searching for over half an hour in my icy temple. Slowly I stood up and watched as droplets of water ran down my torso and fell back in to the bath. All this seemed to be happening in slow-motion. A few moments later I saw steam rising up off my arms and shoulders. By now I was use to the temperature. I stepped out of the bath and on to a cold linoleum floor. The temperature outside was roughly six degrees. In my bathroom, naked and wet, it was considerably colder.

My train of thought shifted to how my body could function in this extreme condition that I had put myself in. It was probably warmer in my fridge at the time. I also pondered on the fact that my autonomic nervous system kept me alive while I slept. So presumably there must be a part of my brain that dealt with temperature control. It would just take time to kick in that's all. I was fascinated to see how long. That's a typical Gemini trait of mine. I stepped into the hallway and sat down on the pine flooring.

I didn't dry myself or get dressed. I waited until I dried off naturally. After the cold temperature in the bathroom the hall felt comparatively warmer. It was only a few degrees' difference but it registered immediately. I was completely dry in about half-an-hour, the experience was most fore-filling. I felt I had humbled myself enough, as a reward I wrapped a huge white towel round my shoulders. I sat there for ages soaking up the priceless sensation of warmth and well-being. Socks were my first item of clothing that I put on. Once I was dressed, I could fully appreciate the material on my skin.

I went and lay down on a mattress I had on the front room floor. I stared into space without blinking for so long I could see liver spots moving across my eyes. This kept me amused for quite some time, watching all manor of ghost like figures moving like jellyfish. I was frightened to shut my eyes in case I ruined the view of my personalised psychedelic film. Of course I did blink eventually but thankfully the film show continued. Only now the translucent blobs started to get bigger and began to change colour. My eyes had become a projector and the front room wall was the screen, which was now a swirling mass of red and blue neon's. I lay there totally transfixed as a whole array of patterns appeared in front of me.

Rather than worrying why this was happening I went with it. At one point the neon's looked like two shoals of fish that had been disturbed by a predator. It was a truly amazing sight as I watched the patterns change time and time again. The coloured neon's began to slow down and I presumed that this was the end of the film. They came to a halt and I could make out a face, in the style of Salvador Dali. I was stunned to see on closer inspection that it was a huge picture of my dad. I felt water running down my cheeks it was lovely to see him this way and, deep, deep inside my head I could hear his voice saying, "Try not to worry too much son, it will all turn out okay in the end." It wasn't until that moment that I realised just how much I missed being called son.

This perfect scene was soon to be shattered with the return of the helicopter. To add to the noise pollution I heard the return of people running through the flats still screaming. I heard the internal door to the flats squeak open, then crash into the brickwork behind it. Followed by what sounded like a herd of elephants charging up to the third floor landing. On their way back down the intruders seemed as if they jumped on each step individually, ending up outside my front door. I only had one thought running through my mind at the time, self-preservation.

My place was surrounded it seemed and I had to find some means of protecting myself from these faceless foes. I dragged a large roll of carpet from a back bedroom and placed it a foot away from the front door, and then I poured methylated spirits all over it. I made a liquid trail down the hallway back to where the front room door used to be. I had a heavy curtain hanging up to keep the draft out. I pulled it down and drenched it with water. After hanging it back up I put the half filled meth's bottle in the centre of the hall and then returned to the front room. I opened the window and looked down to see I had a thirty-foot drop onto grass, less if I had time to climb out and drop from my hands.

The plan was simple. As the door was smashed in it would knock over the carpet roll this intern would hit the Meth's bottle at which point I could ignite the Meth's trail and whoosh up it goes. This would give me enough time to escape out of the front room window. I sparked up my Zippo, crouched down near the water logged curtain waiting for God knows what to come bursting through my door. The infernal noise was still growing in volume outside and the helicopter was still flying round and round. My heart was banging against my chest. Sweat was pouring down my face and all my senses where now fully engaged. The helicopter made yet another swoop above the flat; the noise was so intense at this point I felt as though my head was going to explode. Then just as I thought I couldn't take it any more it went quite as a grave yard. The silence was deafening and I felt my heart rate begin to drop. The only things I could hear now were two birds calling to each other. It was starting to get light. This was the first daylight I remember seeing in three days. My nightmare was finally over, or was it..?

To this day I have no recollection of what happened next. However, later on I discovered that the police were keeping tabs on me and at one point I managed to lose them for six hours. I don't know where I went or what I did. The people running through the flats it seems were partygoers. The helicopter wasn't a figment of my imagination but it wasn't following me that night. The garage scenario was a real event.

CHAPTER TEN

<<<< HEALTH, WEALTH & BACK IN THE SLAMMER >>>>

In the early part of 1997 health wise at least, things were going well. I met a new partner, Barbara and within a few short months I had moved in with her and her three children Daniel, Jamie and Bill. After the coldness of my flat, it felt good to be somewhere with a family atmosphere. I even rose to the dizzy heights of full-time employment again. For a brief period I was able to forget I had a serious illness.

After a couple of weeks had past by I told the foreman and the blokes in my department that I was a care in the community statistic. They all seemed genuinely unfazed by my revelation and were all very supportive. At last everything was going my way again. That is until our boss wanted to introduce a new shift system. I could see my near future unravelling like a huge ball of twine. By now most print firms, both small and large, had a day, an evening and a night shift. This was due too strong competition from companies abroad. For the first month everything was fine. There wasn't so much pressure on me unlike my last shift job. But unfortunately the change from day work to late's and early's, a week about, altered my eating and sleeping pattern again. It was only a matter of time before I had my fourth breakdown.

Barbara, who like many people new nothing about a bipolar high was about to experience one, from start to finish, as a carer. This would test our new relationship to its fullest extent. By comparison this breakdown wasn't that bad. But as before it cost me an income, led me back to hospital and put me back into the benefits system. I'll spare you most of the details of my fourth breakdown at the risk of repeating myself. This chapter is really for first time carers like Barbara. It highlights the problems she faced and the lengthy process of my readmission to a psychiatric ward. Let the abridgement begin…

I'm not too sure of the order of things that lead to my dismissal from work. First I had a job and then I seemed to be spending a lot of time at home. I can just recall getting the 'strange looks' part of the illness. Day by day Barbara noticed the odd things that I did, like making sure the fridge magnates were all in perfect alignment. She also saw the changes in my character as I became slowly higher. This situation was only going to get worse for her. In these early stages of my illness Barbara used to have a full-time job and didn't know what she was going to come home to.

One of the first things I did was to pull down the kitchen curtains and throw them out of the window. Then I decided to clean the windows with neat bleach. When a neighbour asked if I was doing a spot of spring-cleaning I said, no we're having some new curtains delivered. Blatant lying can mask a high episode for months on end. Barbara arrived home to find her curtains in the front garden and an opaque frosting on the kitchen windows where the bleach had dried in the sun. She wasn't impressed. Mind you, once she washed off the residue of bleach with a sponge and hot water the windows sparkled for months!

The next day I decided it would be a great idea to crawl across the work-surfaces and draining board with a ten-inch carving knife in my mouth. Having received my Cub Scout badge for safety, I thought it wise to grip the knife in my teeth with the blade edge facing away from the sides of my mouth. It's as just as well I did because I slipped off the worktop. As I smashed to the floor I hit my ankle, hip, elbow and the left hand side of my head. Fortunately as I hit the deck, the knife became dislodged from my mouth and bounced away from my body.

My fantasies were low key by comparison but I still had them on a daily basis. I had a spate of non-arrestable offences and went on spending sprees. I was also hearing voices in my head of people I knew. I had a couple of incidences in pubs, one where I was barred and the other where the police were called out but no arrest was made. As my high gathered momentum Barbara noticed a vast change in my personality. The situation had long past the interim funny stage and hit the 'what the fuck do I do now' stage. Barbara phoned my mum. Shortly after the call mum came over and stayed for a couple of weeks to give some much needed moral support.

On my next outing the stakes rose to the point where I became a public nuisance. It was at this stage that I could be arrested under the mental health act. This was Barbara's only hope of a break from my antics. I had driven from Tottenham to Chingford aiming for my old drinking hole. The pub was situated bang opposite my repossessed bricks and mortar. I was held in different conversations throughout the evening, but they all seemed to finish with people walking away frowning. I honestly didn't have a clue that I was upsetting their feelings. In my high state plus the alcoholic intake my brain must have converted my retorts to peoples' conversation into smart arse replies. I felt the mood around me change when I growled, "I don't give a monkeys, I want to finish my drink first."

A hand reached across from behind me and relieved me of my pint. Some words were uttered in my right ear and shortly after that my left hand made a rendezvous between my shoulder blades. There were some colourful exchanges of language and then I was helped to the floor by an unknown assailant. My next recollection was of being in the same position only now I was outside on the concrete at the front of the pub. From my resting point I saw the familiar sight of a flashing blue light bouncing off the brickwork of the surrounding buildings. The whole evening seemed to be a series of five minute interludes that I remember, and five minutes of amnesia. I don't remember how or why but now I was at the back of the pub in the beer garden. I was sitting down at bench and someone behind me had their arms around my chest and arms. In front of me were four police officers, three male and one female. I could see their lips moving but as before I heard no sound. Obviously this stymied the talking down process but they weren't to know that I couldn't hear them. By all accounts I made it clear that I didn't want a free ride in their nice white van. What I did want was my missing pint back. I was seriously pissed off about that and started taking out my wrath on the officers present. I began lashing out with a series of karate style side kicks with my left leg. This gave the boys and girl in blue all the ammunition they needed to wade in and arrest me.

After another memory lapse I found myself sitting astride a low wall at the front of the pub in plod bracelets. Shortly after that the back doors of the police van were shut behind me. Someone from the pub, I never found out who, phoned Barbara to make her aware of the situation and where I was. This news came as a great relief to her. At last someone was in a position to give me the help I needed and the rest she wanted. Unfortunately her breathing space was short lived. Our destination, although I didn't know it at the time, was a psychiatric unit called, Naseberry court. I remember clocking the sign on the building and thinking, this isn't Claybury and I was right, it wasn't. Claybury had closed its doors for the last time in 1999 when it was sold off to developers. The reason the name rang a bell was because it was the name of a ward in the hospital. But I digress. I was handed over to a man in a white coat for an assessment of my mental stability.

Initially I was questioned in a small office by two male nurses. Ten minutes later we were joined by two more male members of staff. Soon after they had sat down a fifth male nurse entered the ever shrinking room. I must admit I felt a little under dressed; I was the only one without a white coat! Approximately 40 later minutes I convinced the straitjacket gang that I was well enough to be released back into the wild. God knows how, not only was I on a high I was also five pints to the wind. I can only assume that once I had calmed down the alcohol in my system put me on some sort of automatic pilot. The general public's view would be, how is it possible for a person to be cross questioned by five trained professionals and then sent home? I can just imagine the headlines in the tabloids if I had gone off on one, "NUTTER SET FREE." All joking aside I know how difficult it is to prognosticate an individual high episode.

The only question I can clearly recall was being asked to sign a piece of paper on a clipboard at the end of the meeting. In light of what had happened at the pub, my trip in the fuzz wagon and where I was at the time, my immediate response was, "I'm not signing anything until I'm sitting in a cab on my way home." A car was called for. True to my word I signed the relevant paperwork through the open window of the taxi. The driver looked most perturbed at this situation. I arrived home in Tottenham at 12-15pm. Both Barbara and my mum looked at me in utter disbelief at my appearance. They felt sure or were hoping at least that I would be kept in over night, if only for observational purposes. It wasn't to be, well not this night anyway. Barbara looked absolutely shattered through worry and lack of sleep. I had been on the loose, high and still able to drive for over four weeks.

It came to a point where Barbara had to call out the emergency doctor. On this particular night I had been rolling around on our bedroom floor saying that I felt as if my head was going to explode. That same night I also had an uncontrollable manic laughing fit that lasted over an hour. This was the last straw. She was petrified. All Barbara could do was watch me go through this awful ordeal until the locum arrived.

Around 2-30am there was a tap on our door. At last, Barbara had some physical evidence that she wasn't fighting this battle by herself anymore. I heard some mumbled conversation emanating from our kitchen. Minutes later a nervous looking middle aged man entered our bedroom clutching his box of tricks. We chatted for a while about the usual stuff. How was I feeling in myself and how was my diet and sleep pattern? I couldn't answer the first two questions, but the third one was a doddle. I replied, "I was training to be an undercover driver for the police and I train at night, anyway, sleep's for poofs! You know what; I don't think he believed me!

The usual attempt was made to get me back in hospital but it failed. The doctor offered me an injection and I told him where he could stick it. However I did accept his third option which was the large red tablet. He explained to Barbara that this drug would knock me out and calm me down. It didn't. He left and so did the three coppers who were hovering on the stairs. After two hours sleep I woke up raring to go again. Barbara had been in the same helpless situation now for five weeks. She felt she had been deserted by the very people who should have been able to end this nightmare. Barbara was left asking herself the same question she had been asking herself for the last 35 days. What does it take to get an ex inpatient back through the hospital doors?

A day or two later the hospitals front line trooper arrived in the shape of the head psychiatrist. I wasn't interested in a thing he had to say. I was more intent in playing my music as loud as possible. Through the noise I refused his

184

invitation of a comfy bed, three square meals a day and all the tablets I could get down my face. He left empty handed. Barbara was left with tears and tiredness again. There must have been a lull in high state because I agreed to a consultation with my GP. I began taking my medication again, 800 Mg of Lithium carbonate and an anti-depressant of a 100 Mg per day. In a couple of weeks I began to feel calmer but I didn't feel right in myself. I was forgetful, confused and disorientated at different times of the day. In this pliable state I also agreed to a meeting with the head shrink that visited the house. More drugs were prescribed, Haliperidol and Valium four times a day. With the cocktail of drugs I was now taking I slipped into vegetative state. I was like that for a fortnight. In that time I had an allergic reaction to the Haliperidol and revisited the wonderful world of akathisia. Not the sit down get up variety. This strain of the side-effect made it impossible for me to lie down for more than two seconds at a time.

My run back into hospital was more of an implosion rather than the expected explosion. One Sunday afternoon a relative of Barbara's dropped in to see how we were. Me, I was totally out of the game. I couldn't string a sentence together at the time. Even though I was sitting down I had the sensation that I was floating. It was even worse when I closed my eyes or walked about. Barbara well, she had played the watching and waiting game now for seven long weeks and was absolutely shattered. As the two talked over their tea I sat in silence with a blank expression on my face. To get my full attention Barbara's cousin sat on my lap and asked me how I was. I looked around the room then up at her and said, "I think I should go to hospital now." I don't think Barbara knew whether to laugh or cry first. Either way I could see the look of relief in her tired eyes.

When the ward doctor read through my medical notes he remarked, "No, no this can't be right, who told you to take all of these drugs together?" "My doctor and the head shrink." I replied. Clearly the two doctors had got their wires crossed with regard to who was giving me what in the drug department. I was no longer high anymore, that was the good news, and the bad news was that I had been over medicated for the last14 days. Perhaps they misread my medication notes, who knows? Either way the after effects of this dropped bollock cost me six months of usual living. After a week of detox I was discharged.

When I returned home I lived like a recluse. The only reason to venture outside was for cigarettes. I found myself hiding in the bathroom or the bedroom to get away from the noise generated by Barbara's three boys. It was even worse in the school holidays especially the summer break. That was six weeks of hell for me. Eventually the symptoms I had from the medication mix up did fade away. I think it took about three months for my ears to settle down. A month after that I was able to peeled my first potato. The drugs in my system at the time had made all my finger joints swell up so much I couldn't hold a knife and fork.

I returned to hospital for monthly check ups and blood tests for my Lithium levels. It was there that I was informed that my social interactive skills were falling short of the mark. Whose fault was that? The suggestion was made that I should attend the hospitals' day care plan. This meant change. I didn't like change. I still don't. I immediately erected as many barriers in my thought compartment to thwart this scheme getting off the ground. "I can't use public transport at the moment. We don't have a car and I can't afford to get a cab everyday." All of which was true but this is why the care plan had been introduced. The doctor's reply knocked over my fences in one sentence. "That's not a problem, I will arrange for the hospital mini bus to pick you up." I only had one more fence left, "I can't get up in the morning because my sleep pattern is still broken." "Oh I'm sure your wife will make sure you're up in time won't you Mrs. Walton?" Barbara nodded and smiled in agreement. This was going to be an awful experience, I couldn't remember the last time I saw two eight o'clocks in the same day.

When the first week was over I convinced myself I didn't want to return on the following Monday. The first part of the day was spent in the music therapy room. We were each asked to bring in a piece of music that we liked by the nurse taking the session. Once the record, tape or CD had finished playing we had to comment on why enjoyed our choice of song. When you feel like you don't like anything conversation is sparse. You feel such a prat when you open your mouth and nothing comes out. It was an uncomfortable experience to begin with; made worse by the fact that there were fifteen sets of unknown eyes all focusing their attention on you. We all had or gave a reaction to the music that was played, even if it was only nervous laughter. My main thoughts were, thank fuck it's not my turn yet and goodness is it tea time already I'll miss my go.

I found the questions and answers session the most helpful. I got a chance to vent my own feelings and listen to people in a similar situation as myself. I also got to find out more about my medication which I desperately needed to do at the time. It's bad enough having an invisible condition. But it's even harder trying to explain the invisible side-effects of your medication to your partner. I got to the point where even I thought I was making it up. This part of the day proved to be the most beneficial. I was getting what I needed finally, concrete information.

We broke for lunch at 12pm, well everybody except me that is. I was still in a fragile state and suffering from acute anxiety attacks. Standing in the queue was like strap hanging in a full tube train carriage. I couldn't deal with the confinement of a narrow corridor and broke out in an all over sweat. After ten minutes the canteen doors were opened and the muttering crowd ambled forward. Then came the horrendous sound of clattering china on plastic trays, both of these items were slammed down onto a steel work-surface and cutlery dropped on all of the above. To add to this percussive ensemble, there were people pushing, queue jumping and a chorus of screams and arguments. No, no, no, no, no, I wasn't prepared to put myself through that. I side stepped lunch for two weeks.

The last session of the day was aromatherapy using various oils and creams. Personally I couldn't see the point of this perfumed pastime. You have to bear in mind that there were people in different stages of recovery. Some were further off their trolley than I was and that included the person taking the session! She was a jolly hockey sticks kind of a gal, if you no what I mean. I caught her having long conversations with herself on more than one occasion. In fact when she turned up for the first time I thought she was a patient! There's more out than in you know. Hmmm, makes you think doesn't it...

In no time at all people started slapping pungent lotions on their hands, arms and necks. I just sat and watched. On this particularly hot and sunny day combined with the day rooms heating system, it didn't take to long for the oxygen to leave the room. I felt like reaching and left to follow it. When I returned to my seat one of the patients had rolled his shirt up to his chin. He was using his stomach as makeshift palate for different creams. As he weighed thirty stone plus his palate did runneth over. By the end of the session he smelt like a tarts' handbag. I have to say aromatherapy didn't do it for me, I couldn't see how a smell would make me feel any better. I managed to avoid the smell-arama period by slipping out of a side-door or hiding in the toilets before the session started. The hospital bus picked us up at three o'clock. I arrived home shattered, starving and smelling like I had been in a one star bordello all afternoon.

I stayed with the day care plan for two months and things did change for me. I was eating and sleeping at the right time of day and my social skills improved also. But I did get to a stage where I wasn't getting anything out of it and began missing the odd day here and there. To be honest with you it made a nice change to by myself. I was discharged after three months and put in touch with, Hilary who was an occupational therapist at a local mental health unit.

After weeks and weeks of meetings with her slowly but surly some of my self esteem and confidence began to return. She asked me to consider starting a beginners' computer course. It was free and close to the health unit. The usual thoughts crossed my mind. I will fail, I will feel stupid, I will break something, and I won't be able to find the place, even if it is only around the corner and countless others. It was time to put down the stick that I was beating myself to death with on a daily basis. This was going to be a big step for me. But if I hadn't taken it I would still be going around in the same small circle that I was when I first met Hilary. It meant facing the outside world again, using public transport and talking to complete strangers. Thankfully help was at hand every step of the way. Hilary came with me to the library and introduced me to the lady who ran the course. Prior to this a colleague of Hillary's came with me to make sure I new the bus route. After these prepared steps all I had to do was walk into a room full of strangers and sit in front of a machine I knew nothing about. Piece of cake!

The tutor gave me a rundown of the computers' capabilities. It would have been quicker to list what it couldn't do. She then gave me a brief outline of the keyboards use other than typing. It was clear to me after five minutes that this machine had a far better memory than I did. I was also told that I wouldn't retain much of the information imparted to me on the first day and she was right. The minute Bhvani moved away from my desk I went completely blank. She set up the PC so I could begin typing, before leaving me to it she said, "Just play with it for now and if you get stuck I won't be to far away."

I couldn't type, and I didn't know what to type even if I could which I couldn't, you can see the dilemma I was facing. If I pressed a key by mistake something would go wrong and it did. But hey, if you don't make a mistake you don't make anything. Eventually I typed up a family tree. It took me over an hour to knock out nine lines with two fingers but I did it and felt dead chuffed with myself. I stayed with the course for six months going twice a week. During that time I acquired a small computer from a friend and I was able to practise at home. Hilary was pleased for me. Thanks to her patient coaxing I was now computer literate and I could type, something that I thought I would never be able to do.

At one of our meetings I gingerly mentioned to her that I was thinking of writing a book. I asked her to read the notes from chapter eight where I was beaten by the military police. I was embarrassed to stay in the room with and went outside for a smoke. When I returned, somewhat hesitantly, I expected to find her rolling around on the carpet in fits of laughter at my attempted scrawl. It was all in capital letters and had only full stops for punctuation. Putting down the last page she said, "Let's get you published first." I couldn't believe that someone would take me seriously.

Hilary referred me to another mental health unit called, The Calrendon centre. There among other activities such as art classes, jewellery courses and a fully equipped digital recording studio was an editorial group called, Equilibrium. They still produce a quarterly news letter covering all aspects of mental health issues in the borough of Haringey. The first person I met was the facilitator,

Julia Bard. As the group were half through producing their next edition Julia asked me if I wouldn't mind sitting in for now just to see how things ran. I said, no, that's fine I already felt out of my depth and wondered if I should look for the nearest bus stop. She assured me that everything would be fine and took me to meet the rest of the team.

I had spent the last ten years under the crushing power of my fluctuating condition, thinking I would never amount to anything ever again. But here sat a group of mental health survivors being trained by a professional and actually creating something worthwhile. It was a real positive eye opener for me. The groups' illnesses ranged from clinical depression through to schizophrenia. And, despite their respective conditions they all still had a lot of fight left in them. With their inspiration and Julia's positive encouragement the writing was on the wall. All I had to do was transfer my scribbled beginnings from the brickwork to a piece of papyrus and at some point in the future I may be able to call myself a writer. Amongst them I felt sheepish and vastly out of place and said as much. But the internal humour of the illness came forth with a quotation from, Geoff one of the groups writers. "Your not out of place your in a position to give something back, and as long as you're barking mad and can write your own name, you're in!" I was, I could and I'm still there…

At the end of the session I mentioned to Julia that I was toying with the idea of writing a book about being diagnosed with my disorder. This would be the acid test verdict I needed to hear. By comparison Hilary's comments were a tester. Julia was a fully-fledged journalist with years of experience under her belt, what she said now could effect the next five years of my life. I sat back in my chair and waited for an eruption of laughter followed by a 'there there' pat on the head. Julia's concise reply was, "That's a great idea, strong subject too, have you brought any of your work in with you?" I hadn't. At that stage what I had scribed was still in note form. It was written in long hand and minus its paragraphs. AnD My spellinge and punkchewation was orfull!?! "It didn't matter." Julia said. Luckily me grammar posed know problems at all! "Bring what you have so far, she said, and the group can edit it down and we will make it part of the next edition." Well slap me with a four pound trout, that was the first time that I had heard my scribblings described as work. I had no reason not to carry on writing. This was one of those pinpoint days of my life, like where were you when the twin towers collapsed? It was 12.15pm on Friday the 14th of May 1999.

In the coming weeks I began to feel useful and inspired again. My confidence and self-esteem returned to a point where even I noticed a difference in myself. For anybody suffering from depression this is a landmark plateau of their recovery. At my own pace I learnt how to write articles and even attempted some poetry. Three months later I saw my name in print for the first time. I was to see it again when the group and Julia agreed to print part of my book that I had written on E.C.T. On the 9/10/99 Barbara and I got married. This was turning out to be the best year on record since my illness began back in 1989.

To improve my spelling and punctuation Julia made a suggestion that I should consider taking an English language course. Me, in college? It sounded like something other people did. You know 'well' people. That was my brains first depression riddled message. But the more I thought about this challenge the more I wanted to take it on. My illness had given me this time, this hole in my life, not everybody gets this chance to re-educate themselves and undertake the mammoth task of writing their first book. In September 2000 I began my English course at The College of North East London. In the summer of 2001 an envelope dropped on the mat. I was now the proud owner of a piece of paper that stated that I had passed my GCSE exams with 'C' and 'B' grades. Not bad for a forty-three year old bloke with a mental health history as long as both of your arms! It was a strange twist in my fate line in many ways. Without 'my' bipolar disorder I wouldn't have met the people who helped shape and develop my new life altering talent – and you wouldn't be reading this.

I have always had a dominant creative side to my character, I just didn't realise it when I was a child. When I was growing up I was laughed at by my social circle, and this is what I would hear on a daily basis. "That's a stupid idea." "That's a waste of time." "You're mad." And, "Only you could dream up something like that Walton." I have been fighting against this patronisation all of my life. I now feel that it was only a matter of decades before a mental disorder found me. This in turn radically altered my equilibrium and put me on the path that I was destined for.

I had a good run of health from the end of 1998 to the middle of 2002. But the illness being what it is always seems to be lurking around the corner for me. After completing the morning school run I sat down with a mug of tea to see what the Kilroy Silk programme had to offer. The subject that day was about women who suffered with depression. I watched with bated breath hoping to hear if there would be a similar programme scheduled for the male populous. At the end of the show Kilroy announced just that, and a phone number came up on the screen. Before the credits had finished I rang the show and left my name and phone number. At 2.30 the same day the phone rang and Barbara answered it. "Sorry, did you say the Kilroy Silk programme; hold on you'll want to speak to my husband."

CHAPTER ELEVEN

<<<< THIS IS THE BBC >>>>

I was pottering around in the kitchen at the time; I knew who it was before Barbara picked up the phone. Putting her hand over the receiver she said excitedly, "Come on it's somebody from the Kilroy show, hurry up, when did you phone them?" With a knowing smile, possibly smug, I replied, "This morning while you were out."

I had kept quiet about my call to the programme because I had said things in the past and got those looks you get when someone thinks you've missed your medication. Which I can understand but you end up doubting your hopes and capabilities. Barbara gave me the, 'oh know' glances when I said I wanted to write to Spike Milligan and begged the question, why? In short because I bloody wanted to. I have long admired his groundbreaking humour and own over 45 double cassette comedy programmes from the BBC Radio tape collection; seventy percent of which are Goons episodes. Point two, we shared the same illness. Point three, we were both musicians. Point four, I new a policeman who suffered at the hands of the Goons japery whilst on his beat which past a hotel they were staying in. Point five, I once new Peter Sellers' son, Michael, that was the nearest I had ever been to a Goon. All of this information went into a two page letter which I sent to Mr. Milligan's' agent, Norma Farnes.

Spike wrote back to me a month later thanking me for my correspondence.

I spoke to a programme researcher called, Anne. She cut straight to the chase asking me a long list of personal and direct questions. These ranged from my suicide attempt and what caused it, my hospital admissions and about my medication. Anne then asked if she could speak to Barbara. This was to verify who I was and what I had said about myself was fact not fiction. The last thing I heard Barb say before handing the phone back to me was, "I think this is something he's got to do." Anne apologised for the double checking, I said, "No no, that's fine, after all you don't want some nutter turning up on the set do you?" "Oh very funny," She replied sarcastically. "I can see you and I are going to get along just fine. Well you seem to be the type of person we're looking for, would you like to appear as a guest on the show?" "Wild horses couldn't stop me." I replied. "Great, I've booked you a place and car will pick you up at one o'clock on Wednesday, I'll speak to you then."

When I put the phone down I said to Barbara, "Guess who's going to be on telly then? No photos please I haven't got an agent yet!" I got that look that said, PRAT. I received a similar glance when I said, "I'm just popping round the shop to get a half ounce of Old Shag, see if I've made the nationals and greet my public!" I had forty-eight hours to kill before arriving at the Elstree Studios in Borehamwood. I couldn't wait. The day arrived and so did a driver. In no time at all we were there. Once I had past through the BBC's security check-point I was shown into the Kilroy hospitality suite. My immediate concern was finding somewhere to smoke. An usher directed me to a side-room. Picking up a cup of tea I headed for the smokers' den. There I met some of the other guests and it didn't take long for a conversation to break out. There was a real buzz about the place as I'm sure you can imagine.

Names were being called out, researchers were checking that all of the guests had arrived and we kept looking around to see if we could spot anybody famous. One by one we were given our seat numbers. I didn't know until that moment that I would be sitting in the front row. The buzz that was had just turned into a loud hum as we were led towards the Kilroy set. Before the recording commenced the floor manger gave us a briefing and microphones were clipped to our clothing. At this point we still hadn't seen the show's host. A few minutes later the programmes producer informed us that in sixty seconds the cameras would start rolling. There was an apprehensive hush on set and then Mr. Silk appeared from behind the scenery. He walked down the stairs towards me sat down and talked to the audience for 15 minutes before the debate got underway.

The programme was entitled 'My father committed suicide.' It featured people whose parents had committed suicide and a section of us who had attempted it. In the centre of the stage sat others who couldn't understand why anyone would contemplate killing themselves. Before we new it the title music was playing and we were clapping and saying good morning to Robert Kilroy Silk. This felt really bizarre as it was now three in the afternoon. Not only that usually he's standing inside a small flashing coloured box in the corner of our living room!

The debate opened with a man whose father had killed himself, right from the start he was sobbing poor bloke. We later learned that his father had hung himself because of mounting debts within his family run business. It was David, his son who found him. This painful event had ruined his marriage and the majority of his adult life. Some speakers felt that suicides such as these were acts of pure selfishness, especially where children were involved. I disagreed saying, "That's the last thing on your mind." All you want to do is get out of the mental agony you're in."

Drawing from my own experiences I tried to explain what drives a person to commit suicide. One lady in the audience felt responsible for her husbands' death. This is the point where the stick that the sufferer used to beat themselves with gets past onto the next of kin. In reality there was nothing she could have done to stop him. If a person reaches that low ebb they'll just go off and do it. I went on to explain how difficult it was to identify depression, especially in yourself. Appearing on the show felt completely natural and I wasn't nervous at all. Ironically at the time I couldn't use public transport because of the crowds and confinement. But I felt fine in front of four cameras and 80 complete strangers in the studio! After the filming, Kilroy shook my hand, thanked me for coming on the show and said, "I thought you came across very well."

After two and a half hours of debate we were led back to the green room for a well- earned drink. I grabbed two cups of tea and headed straight for the smoking area.

Several members of the audience came over to speak to me and thanked me for what I had said during the show. I left the set feeling as though I had helped a few people understand what depression is like as an illness. If I get the chance again I would like to repeat the experience. At six o'clock I was informed that my driver, 'ark at me, my driver, was waiting to take me back to reality.

Before I left the studio I asked when the show would be aired. I was told that all of the guests would receive a phone call two days prior to the transmission. The programme was recorded on the 30/1/02. It was a great start to my year. It's a shame my good fortune didn't last. Eight weeks had past by and still no phone call. I knew the show would be broadcast it was just a case of being patient. When the call came I was out. Barbara's' eldest son, Daniel took the message one Friday afternoon. Three and a half months after the filming had taken place I could now do the ring round to family and friends.

I wasn't high at the time but my mood was definitely elevated. I put this down to the excitement of being seen on national prime-time television. It had been roughly two years since my last break-down. Somewhere a long the line I had slipped up with the daily intake of my drugs. This is not something I do on purpose. Over the course of two months I had probably halved my medication, so it would be difficult to determine when or if I would go high.

The night before my television debut I had a massive panic attack. I have never experienced anything like it in my life. I was sweating, I felt sick and breathless, my ears were pounding and I found it hard to swallow. As I stood up from my chair I felt a tremor in the pit of my stomach. All of a sudden, whoosh it was as if I had a tornado raging in my guts. It swirled around my intestines, bounced off my rib cage and then headed for my skull at the speed of an express train. I really thought the top of my head was coming off. This all happened within a split second of standing up. The locomotive came to a halt using my brain as a buffer. I said to Barbara in a panic, "Tablets, I need to take my tablets." She asked me how I felt and what did I want to do? As I bent over the kitchen sink trying to compose myself I replied, "I think I'd better go and get checked out."

We arrived at St. Anne's a little after eight in the evening. I gave the receptionist my details and after a nail biting wait I was called into a room by a female doctor. I explained what had happened at home and I also mentioned that I thought I had missed some of my medication. She then asked me what was going on in my life at the moment. Have you ever opened your mouth and wished you hadn't? Baring in mind where I was, why I was there and who I was talking to I replied, "Well I'm writing a book and tomorrow morning I'm going to be on television." As soon as I opened my gob I thought she's never going to buy that last bit.

"Okay," She said. "How do you feel at this very moment?" "Well, (and here comes my full mental check list) I do feel a little confused but I know where I am and everything around me is real. I'm not hearing voices. I don't feel aggressive, nobody is trying to put thoughts into my head and I can't control other people's minds. I'm not having fantasies or hallucinations either, my diet is okay and my sleep pattern is better than it used to be I just feel odd." I could only assume that I had the panic attack because I had bollocksed up my drug quota. I think I looked how I felt - vacant. After an in depth line of questioning lasting over thirty minutes the doctor now wanted to speak to Barbara. I was glad of the break to be honest with you. My heart was pounding and my face felt as if it had a fire-hearth glow about it. I went outside to cool down and caught up on some smoking. Barbara was in with the doctor for as long as I was. Eventually she came out to me and said that the doctor wanted to speak to both of us. If nothing else the hospitals' procedure for my check up was thorough.

The doctor spent a considerable time going over the main points of the interview. This allowed Barbara an opportunity to verify or deny my answers. Even the doctor saw the funny side of things when I mentioned my television appearance. I had escaped an over night stay in hospital due to the fact that I had been taking some of my medication and my speech was lucid throughout my check up.

I was pleased that Barbara had an involvement with my interview; after all it would be her that copped the initial front-line flak if my health deteriorated any further. The doctor went on to say, "So if your wife is happy with what's been said you can go home, just make sure you start taking your correct amount of medication. If you are in any doubt come straight back." We left the hospital feeling mentally drained arriving home shortly after quarter to eleven.

The next day I was woken up with a nudge, a mug of tea and the sound of the Kilroy signature tune coming from our bedroom television. I grabbed my cigarettes, sat up and watched the whole sixty-minute show in complete silence. Because of the gap between recording and transmission I had forgotten some of the things that I had said. It also took me a while to adjust to the way I looked and sounded. I was surprised to see so much of me after the programme had been edited down to an hour. I had more than my fifteen minutes of fame quoted by Mr. Warhol. A friend said jokingly, that the camera loved me, and I must admit I did have a lot to say and this was the perfect platform. Overall I thought the subject matter came across well.

When the programme finished, I went outside to catch a breath of fresh air as I was still groggy from the night before. I don't think I had walked more than ten yards when a neighbour spotted me and said, "Was that you I just saw on the Kilroy show?" Fame at last! I nodded and couldn't help smiling. "You poor man." She said. "How do you cope with an illness like yours?" "With the help from a lot of people and blind determination." I replied. With that I toddled off to Sainsburys.

On the way there I was stopped by two complete strangers. To add to this, on my return I was stopped by a young man who had also watched the show. He thought that I was brave to go on the programme and talk so candidly about my experiences with depression. I said I don't know about brave, I just saw it as an opportunity where I might be able to show people that they weren't on there own with this illness. It was a day of coincidence. It turned out that this young chap lived on the same housing estate as I did. We had more to talk about when he informed me that he was suffering from clinical depression. The cherry on that days cake was when he told me he had also appeared on Kilroy, in a show about depression in the under twenties. How spooky is that!

Things started to go down hill health wise shortly after my small screen exposure. Even though I had begun to take my powdered cosh on a regular basis again I think I had reached the point of no return. Barbara was so concerned that she started taking down notes of my antics. I'm glad she did. It nipped this potentially high episode right in the bud rather than let it bloom into a flower of chaos. All the same she still had her hands full with this partial high of mine. Her notes are a perfect example of the early stages of a bi-polar high, documented for someone who has never witnessed one before showing all the classic signs.

BARB'S NOTES

Maybe I'm worrying over nothing but Neil is acting strange. He's been putting things down and forgetting where he has left them, like when he couldn't find the hammer. He's been like it since we went to Judie's Dad's funeral. Now he is only getting five hours sleep a night. The other day he left all his CD's over the front room carpet. Neil never leaves his CD collection out on purpose. 14/6/02

Worried about the money situation, he's paying everything by queue at present. I seem to remember the last time he went high he spent money we didn't have. Perhaps we are better off, and he probably does know what he is doing, and I'm just being paranoid, but I'm not sure. On the next page I'm going to make a list of all the strange things he does and make a note of how many hours he sleeps. I can show this record to someone if anything happens. 17/6/02

1. Says he's not hungry - poor diet

2. Not sleeping - broken sleep pattern

3. Forgetful - memory loss / confused / unable to concentrate

4. Organising things i.e. - Cupboards, drawers, fridge magnets.
   Obsessive behaviour

5. Playing music loud - he says it's therapy / euphoria

SLEEP

*   *
*

Sunday	16/6/02	4 Hours
Monday	17/6/02	5 Hours
Tuesday	18/6/02	7 Hours
Wednesday	19/6/02	4 Hours
Thursday	20/6/02	5 Hours
Friday	21/6/02	Didn't come to bed
Saturday	22/6/02	Didn't come to bed

Sunday   23/6/02   Didn't come to bed 3 hours in evening - awake all night

Monday   24/6/02   5.30pm to 11.45pm. Then awake
all night
Tuesday   25/6/02   7.45pm to 2.30am.   Then awake
all night   - Hospital visit

Wednesday   26/6/02   8.15pm to 1.00am … Then awake
all night
Thursday   27/6/02   Hospital
*   *
*

****** Can days, dates & hours be set better? I've tried
but no joy******
Tonight Neil said that we are going to get some help and
things are things are going to get better, something to do
with the Masons. They're going to help us but without us
knowing. (Fantasising) …   I think all he needs to do is
concentrate on getting better and take his tablets. He also
mentioned that he had a check up with Morris's son who
happens to be a doctor, which he is.   He's trying to
convince me that he is okay and the more he does the more
I doubt him. I don't want to, but I'm watching him take his
tablets again. I'm worried sick. 18/6/02

Well it all started up last night about one in the morning.
He couldn't sleep and was holding his head but kept saying
he was all right. He went downstairs and put some music
on quite loud, lit candles both upstairs and downstairs. At
3am he went out to get a take-away. I came down at 7am
and he wasn't here. I phoned about for him but by twenty
past eight he came back. He said he'd been to the café,
Sainsburys and then for a drive. I asked him if we could

go to the hospital and he said yes but now he's gone upstairs. I'll have to do my best to get him there. I'm so tired and scared, only having had three hours sleep myself. 24/6/02

Went to hospital and the doctor said he was high. He asked Neil if he wanted to stay in but he refused saying we were ganging up on him. (Paranoia) Went outside for a fag and Neil said he would stay in, but then changed his mind. BASTARD. Went home. Managed to get his tablets down him and tonight at 7.45pm, with a full stomach, he has fallen asleep. 25/6/02

Neil slept until 2.30am. I went back to bed at 3am. Went downstairs at 5am cos the dog was barking, Neil had gone out. When I came back down at 7am he was indoors. Ron, a neighbour said he saw Neil at about 6.30am. My alarm goes off at 7.05am so he must have gone out twice. EVENING: Well he hasn't disappeared around the pub like last night. Chris, the landlady came and got me, she said he was talking to himself. I caught him a couple of times but if you say anything he says he thought he heard me ask him something. 26/6/02

At 5am we had tai chi in the garden and a lot of banging on the fence. He told the boys that he had passed a tai chi exam (It doesn't exist) and he's going to get a certificate. He also said that Judie, his ex wife, had put him up for some sort of award. (No she hadn't) This was filmed at 6am this morning in Sainsburys car park. (Fantasy) Hopefully he'll sleep a little longer than last night, even half an hour would be nice, I'll let you know in the morning. 27/6/02

Well he slept until 1am on Thursday and seemed to get worse as the day went on. Arrived at the hospital and the doctor could see he wasn't well, he asked Neil if he would stay in and he said yes. When we got over to the ward he told the nurses he didn't want to stay and kicked up a stink. Shortly after that they *Sectioned* him. At first they said he was under a 72 hour Section, then a social worker phoned to say that he might be in for a fortnight or maybe longer. He looks so helpless in there and I feel so guilty that I've left him there. I had to sneak away. All I have done is cry. This morning, as soon as I opened my eyes I cried for him. I know he's in the best place and the nurses seem very nice; even Neil said it was better than Claybury. I told him I love him and we had lots of good kisses. Tonight I just wanted to hold him. I was scared to see him but now I have he seems a lot calmer so I'm glad I went. Now I've got wages to earn and shopping to get plus fags for Neil every day. I'm not going to worry about it at the moment, tomorrow's another day. Please God make him well, he's the best thing in my life apart from the kids and if he takes his tablets we could be so happy together. All this does is tear us up in pieces. Need some sleep, will see him Saturday at 2 o'clock, good night. 28/6/02

When Barbara slipped away I was in the wards' garden going through a speeded up tai chi routine. Every now and again I heard a nurse calling out to inform me that I had to take some medication. On more than one occasion I shouted back, "You're not supposed the take any medication on an empty stomach, even you know that." Of course now I had been sectioned they could administer the drugs by force if necessary. I was coaxed into the ward corridor and very quickly found myself surrounded by six strapping male nurses. Things went blank at this point. I don't recall a struggle or being pinned down on a bed and injected but according to a fellow inmate I was. It's just something that has to be done sometimes.

Within a week I was allowed out on home visits and seemed to be recovering quicker than my previous break-downs. But there always seems to be something that fucks up my progress. The first thing I noticed was that I began to lose my sense of balance. A couple of days later I found myself slurring my words and my tongue was now bigger than the cavity it was supposed to rest in. Then all the muscles in my arms cramped up at once and I was unable to rest them down by my side. My facial colour drained from a healthy pink to a nasty shade of fag ash grey. What ever was causing these symptoms it was getting worse by the day. It had taken roughly 14 days to end up in this debilitating state and I was in a great deal of physical pain. Even my assigned nurse mentioned to Barbara how worried he was about the way I looked.

On day sixteen I was slurring nicely, crippled with pain, off balanced, off colour and now sweating like a welder from the minute I got up. Eventually the ward doctor was called for. After checking my breathing and blood pressure he uttered the words that no patient wants to hear, "I'm sorry to say I don't know what's wrong with you." The words, marvellous, fucking and oh sprang to mind! I was shipped off to another hospital for overnight tests. There, not a lot seemed to be happening. I was put on a drip and waited five hours for a bed, that's all that occurred in 12 hours. The next morning I was taken back to my ward by ambulance still no nearer a cure for my ailments. That night I was standing, or should I say trying to stand, in the queue for medication when I slumped to the floor in agony. The cramp that had invaded the top half of my body had now spread to my legs. It was back to the hospital and back on an overnight drip.

At midday the results of my second set of tests were delivered to the reception desk on the ward. I was surprised to hear that I had had an allergic reaction to my medication. This caused my body to suffer from all of the side-effects known to medical science. Things wouldn't have been so bad if I had only been taking one tablet a night. But no, not me, I was on a whole bunch of drugs, so the cramp, the sweating, the swelling and the agony I was in could be multiplied by seven. The majority of my drugs were altered and my lithium dosage was reduced from 1000mg to 800mg. Which ever drug it was that sparked my chain reaction allergy added an extra four weeks to my stay in hospital. I was discharged from St. Anne's on the 3/9/02 after spending two and a half months on the ward.

I don't know how Barbara coped during that time. Not only did she manage the school runs, the shopping, the washing, the cooking and the bills but she also made time to visit me every day for ten weeks. Thank you my darling, you're one amazing lady and I love you to bits. In the first week of my section I was asleep when Barb came to see me. On a few occasions I asked her to leave because I didn't know what to say to her. I don't think I have cried so much at any one point in my life. Each time she left the ward to go home I felt as if someone had stuck a knife through my heart, it was awful

Now out of hospital I felt a burden to her. While I was away Barbara had adopted a new routine. I on the other hand had lost mine altogether. I was in that limbo state again, not ill enough to be in hospital and not well enough to do anything constructive around the house. I spent the first six weeks at home hiding in our bedroom like a frightened animal. I was fine if everything was quiet but if there was any noise like the kids charging about, the dog barking, the phone ringing or visitors I was off like a rat up a drainpipe. Institutionalisation, you can't beat it! But you do, I have, five times now and if can so can you. The hardest thing I found to come to terms with right from the start of my illness was a humbler existence caused by financial loss.

Things took a downward swoop when I had to be weaned off the diazepam I was taking. The withdrawal effects of this highly addictive drug have always been a painful experience for me. I felt more confused than usual and I couldn't concentrate on anything for more than five minutes at a time. My whole body ached as if I had a flu virus and I felt irritable and moody for eight long weeks. It was time to get my anti-depressant dosage increased. I waited three days before I could get an appointment with my doctor. I waited in the waiting room for an hour because the surgery was full to bursting. Then I had to wait six weeks before my extra 50mg kicked in. I was in physical pain for five months after my discharge date. Now ten months later (8/4/03) everything is pretty much back to how it was before my break-down.

HOW MY BI-POLAR DISORDER AFFECTS ME TODAY

09/06/03 Thankfully I'm still married. Barbara has seen and had to cope with the fallout of two bipolar high episodes and that's enough for any marriage. A third could prove fatal. Many partners may have walked away from this situation. Barbara didn't, she stood by me every step of the way. I can't thank her enough she is quite unique. So here's a few promises Barb. No more missed medication should equal no more highs and no more hospital admissions.

I'm still unemployed due to my fluctuating illness, which in turn has crushed all my self-confidence in a work environment, but I am hoping to make it as a writer. I have a twelve-year mental health history. I am now forty-six as of the 30/5/03; it doesn't look good on your CV. Some while ago now I heard this quotation from a national employers' survey, "Given the choice employers would rather take on somebody with a criminal record than a person with a mental illness." That was just three years ago. I would like to think that things have changed but I'm not totally convinced. So with regard to a return to full or part time work I think I've got about as much chance of being stabbed by the Pope! Did I mention I'm hoping to earn a living as a writer?

My sleep pattern well, I don't think I'll ever get back on top of that one but it's marginally better than it used to be. This one factor effects everything anybody does so I have to re-jig my day around my sleep pattern. Generally I feel tired all of the time but being lethargic doesn't necessarily mean I'll sleep all through the night. When the kids are at school I have a better routine. Monday to Friday I get up at eight o'clock and after a full English breakfast, two cups of strong tea and five cigarettes, I walk my stepson, Bill to school. When I return home I pull something out of the freezer for the evening meal. The only daytime television I watch is the Kilroy show.

It's now 10am, I've had breakfast and it's time to make a start on the housework. First the kitchen, then the vacuuming and sorting out any washing and drying that needs to be done. At 12 noon I start writing, for two hours usually. If I'm too tired to write during the day I'll do two hours in the evening. By 2pm I have to grab some shuteye, I only had four/five hours sleep the night before and my medication still makes me feel drowsy. This is the nearest I can get to a normal sleep pattern. It also changes according to the weather. I have a better nights sleep during the winter months but it get progressively worse as summer approaches. I don't think I've had a proper nights sleep since my bipolar disorder was diagnosed all those years ago. On Wednesdays I do the weeks shopping and cook six days out of seven. When Friday comes along I meet up with the editorial team of Equilibrium from 10am to 12 noon. On numerous occasions, I have turned up so tired that I couldn't think straight and gave little input to some of the two-hour sessions. But its okay, everybody there is a mental health survivor. So there's no need for a long-winded explanation or guilt, or a crushing blow to your self-confidence that lasts for a week, what I get there is acceptance and understanding without question. At the weekend I can sleep for nine to ten hours and don't need to kip during the day. But come Monday morning me and Mr. Morpheus are at loggerheads again.

Now what else, oh yes, I can't sit in a room full of people for to long, friends or strangers, because I can't filter out the different conversations. I hear everything that is said including what's on the television. Within five to ten minutes I have to leave the room. I head for the kitchen usually, make everyone a cup of tea and then sneak up stairs eventually to the isolation of our bedroom until the noise has subsided. One of Barbs friends took this act personally one day and said I was being anti-social. So I spent the next 45 minutes explaining why I felt the way I did. She still didn't get it. And some feel on stoney ground. A basic school education, it's a wonderful thing in the right hands! I don't like using public transport because of the confinement and noise. I also avoid being surrounded by people I don't know i.e. passengers. This goes back to my second stint in Claybury when I was held down by a group of nurses for the first time and injected to calm me down. Or maybe it was when I was handcuffed and repeatedly beaten when I strayed onto the airfield. Either way I don't like to be near or part of a crowd. My thought process is slow which is embarrassing and frustrating for me, I tend to head for the bedroom if I need to sort a problem out or write a cheque. With regards to going out, I don't like to be to far from home, but at least I leave the house now on a regular basis.

I don't like the fact that the chemicals I have to put in my body control my every action. But there doesn't seem to be anything new available in the drug market. Well nothing that doesn't come with all the usual side-effects. I have taken Lithium and anti-depressants for seven years now and still get some of the side effects attached to my powdered cosh. I have trouble losing weight and I only have to fart and I breakout in a sweat, I don't know why but sweating is embarrassing for me. I seem to have a headache most days, not a migraine, just a dull ache. My mouth is continually dry. This means I drink more and consequently I visit the little boys' room more often than the average male. And the twitch that I have which affects the base of my spine well, I can live with that. Thankfully it's not as pronounced as the one that Jack Douglas has, he of the Carry On films. 'Itch - ch - per – phway' his catch phrase was, just before he threw his pint over someone.

Well this is very nearly the end of my scribblings. I can't believe I have written about 12 years of my life. I hope you have found some of it interesting, or at the very least useful. It's been a bumpy road one way or another, but it did turn out better than I expected. I leave you with two basic pieces of advice and a poem called, Beast of burden, which shows a somewhat accurate view of my day-to-day living. The last bit of advice I can offer is; 'Never ever watch daytime television and keep taking the tablets.'

BEAST OF BURDEN

When I think of what it was to how it is now,
I no longer feel like a sacred cow.

Gone are the days when I'd cower and cry,
Gone are the feelings of wanting to die.

Clear-headed almost and out of my pain,
The light of my tunnel ignited again.

Lost are the feelings of walking on water,
At least I'm not next as a lamb to the slaughter.

But for how long this time?

Neil Walton

23/10/99

THE FIRST THING I EVER WROTE

During the time that Julia Bard was our facilitator at Equilibrium she would set us a writing exercise at the end of each two hour session. Someone would choose a subject and we would write about it. The only proviso was we had a time limit of two minutes. If you couldn't think of anything it didn't matter. You'd be surprised what comes out when you 'free write' as I call it.

This is what I came up with on my first day, word for word in all of its naivety. I arrived feeling inadequate and left enthused and inspired. And it's all thanks to the **Mental Health Services Employment and Training Initiatives**. The Equilibrium editorial team is based in Haringey.

Like-minded people

It's been a long time since I have been in a room full of like-minded people. No questions, just acceptance. I beats therapy, day hospital and talk of medication. It's nice to see other people with a talent and an illness, and not letting that illness mar that talent. At last I feel now I have an outlet for my talent and I have a warm feeling about that...

Neil Walton.   Writing exercise   14 May 1999

Just remember...

There never has been a great talent without a touch of madness.   Seneca

Our greatest blessings come to us through madness.
Socrates

Touch I maybe but brilliant I am.
N Walton

I don't just think outside of the box – I was born outside of the box.   N Walton

ACKNOWLEDGEMENTS

FAMILY & GOOD FRIENDS

Thank you to the following people: my wife Barbara and her family including, Rose, John, Daniel, Jamie and Bill. Also, Ron, Rose and Jackie.

My first wife, Judie and of course my two sons, Jack and Daniel. Also Myrtle and Reg woods, Stan, Rene, Steve, Sue, Simon and Sonia, and Betty and Jerry.

Other credits go to: The Passmores, Joy, Ted, Anne and Bill. Also the Howeth family, Judy, Ron and Seron. And Chris, Lorraine and George.

HEALTH TEAMS AND CARE SPECIALISTS

The staff of the Ridgeway surgery, Chingford. Dr Karen Gibbon, Steve Anderson (CPN). The staff at Claybury Hospital, Dr Gadhvi, Jon Slevin, Trisha and Ian, Roz and Ruma at Quest.

The staff at Morris House surgery, Tottenham. Dr Sally Dowler. All at St. Ann's Hospital, Kate Marsden Unit, including Clare Harris-Evens and Ilene. Also, Hilary

Neals at the Tynemouth Road Centre, who without I wouldn't have begun to write.

THE CLARENDON CENTRE

A special thank you to: Bill Slade, Julia Bard, Maggie Gibbon, Gavin Eastley. Also the Equilibrium editorial team, Antony, Ginny, Pumla and Cassandra. Lastly to my tutor at The College of North East London, Liz Cruse and anyone who I may have forgotten during my various break-downs.

CHIPMUNKA PUBLISHING

Finally I would like to thank the Chipmunka crew for their involvement with this project and Jason Pegler for taking on my 'scribblings.'

THE END

Lightning Source UK Ltd.
Milton Keynes UK
13 May 2010

154127UK00001B/41/A